Mush

from sled dogs to celiac,
the scenic detour of my life

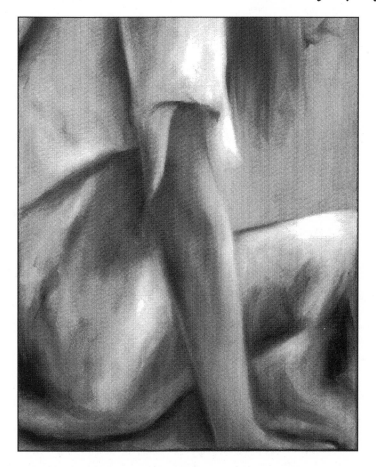

Tara Caimi

Plain View Press
http://plainviewpress.net

1101 W. 34th Street, STE 404
Austin, TX 78705

ISBN: 978-1-63210-005-4
Library of Congress Control Number: 2014942654

Cover painting by Meredith O'Neal
Meredith O'Neal is an expressive oil painter and part-time muralist based in Austin, TX. Through her figurative paintings, she addresses issues of the mind and body. Exploring themes such as intimacy, vulnerability, isolation, and the temporality of humanity, her work can be found at http://www.meredithoneal.com/

Cover photo by Mark Dalmeida at White Mountain Works
White Mountain Works photographs are taken by Mark Dalmeida on his trips and hikes throughout the White Mountains of New Hampshire. He tries to capture moments as naturally and as accurately as possible and to include a story in the description of each piece. White Mountain Works original photography can be found at https://www.etsy.com/uk/shop/WhiteMountainWorks

We Find Healing In Existing Reality
Plain View Press is a 36-year-old issue-based literary publishing house. Our books result from artistic collaboration between writers, artists, and editors. Over the years we have become a far-flung community of humane and highly creative activists whose energies bring humanitarian enlightenment and hope to individuals and communities grappling with the major issues of our time—peace, justice, the environment, education and gender.

for Grammie

This book is a product of memory, not to be confused or equated with fact. Dialogue has been recreated. Names and a few character-defining details have been changed. Some events are combined and timelines shifted to adhere to the relevant storyline.

Mush is a true story, from the author's perspective, as far as she can remember.

Acknowledgments

I am grateful to the editors of the publications in which the following excerpts from *Mush*, or versions thereof, originally appeared:
"Mush" in *The MacGuffin*, 2010; "Sled Team" in *Oh Comely* magazine, 2012; "Without Words" in *Outside In Literary & Travel Magazine*, 2013 and in *Whereabouts: Stepping Out of Place* travel anthology, 2013; "Cat Face" in *Pithead Chapel*, 2013; and "Kayenta" in *Oh Comely* magazine, 2014.

This book would not exist without the Wilkes University Creative Writing Program. Special thanks to Dr. Bonnie Culver and all involved who work without rest to help aspiring writers hear, trust, and share their distinct voices.

I thank my parents, who may not always understand my decisions, but who stand by me as I continue to find my way. They have not only graciously accepted but also generously supported my penchant for sharing the personal details of their lives to enhance my work, and I would not be the writer I am without their support.

Thanks to my early readers for helping to guide *Mush* into the book it became: Tracy Janet, Lauren Wazontek, Kristin Ford, Joan and Frank Porter; my classmates Mary Zbegner and the unforgettable Michael Workstel, whose generosity of spirit lives in all who were lucky enough to have known him.

I am grateful to my summer workshop partner Cindy Simmons, whose unique perspective contributed to the refinement of many individual scenes, and to all the members of my artists group, whose encouragement gave me confidence to move forward and whose intelligence, talent, compassion, and strength continue to awe and inspire me: Elisha Clark-Halpin, Megan Moore, Marisa Eichman, June Ramsey, Elle Morgan, and Meghan Sweeney.

Special thanks to David Stong for reading the manuscript more times than anyone should have to read anything and, as always, for the solid artistic guidance and inspired graphic art and design assistance. Many thanks to Mary Janzen for also repeatedly reading the manuscript and for the linguistic expertise and attention to grammatical detail that helped me look like I know what I'm doing.

I am thankful for the developmental prowess of author Carolyn Turgeon whose advice took the manuscript to another level. I am especially grateful to the editor of *Mush*, Helen Marie Graves, for restoring my faith in my voice and my story and whose thoughtful suggestions guided me toward the light of publication.

Mush may never have seen that light of publication had it not been for the artistic sensibilities of the late Susan Bright, the poet, activist, and founding publisher of Plain View Press, who saw potential in this atypical story of self-discovery. I am thankful to the current publisher of Plain View Press, Pam Knight, not only for honoring Susan's commitment to *Mush* but also for dedicating extra time and attention to help this new author navigate the complexities of the publishing process.

I cannot express the depth of my gratitude to my mentor, the lovely and talented Sara Pritchard. The wisdom and generosity Sara extended— that she embodies and exudes—will stay with me always. I can only aspire to follow the path she has illuminated, to the best of my humble ability.

And finally, to Bill, my partner and my love. I am not worthy, but lucky.

mush:

to embark on a trip or journey, especially over ice or snow with a dog team

a meaningless word, thought to be used as a command to a sled dog team

mawkish sentimentality

a thick porridge

anything unpleasantly lacking in dignity

something thick, soft, and pulpy

Prologue

ON THE SEVENTEENTH DAY of the stomach virus, I rolled off the couch and crawled to the bathroom. I pulled myself up by the sink, wondering what else my body could possibly purge, when the sharpness of a thousand daggers crisscrossing through my abdomen doubled me over in searing pain. A wave of nausea lifted me back up to the sink where I ejected the only food I'd found in the house to eat that day—half of a tuna fish sandwich.

I leaned my now ninety-pound frame into the sink and reached for the spigot. The hand that turned the tap was nothing like my own. Projecting from the weathered skin, spindly bones disguised themselves as fingers with yellowing nails that curled over their tips. I wondered when I had turned eighty. Then I realized that no water was coming out of the faucet. I twisted the handle as far as it could go and reached for the other. Nothing. I heard utility trucks and the sounds of people working in the yard.

You have got to be kidding, I thought as I pushed myself up from the sink, raising my face to the mirror. A thinly veiled skeleton stared back with a vacuous expression. There was no flesh under the skin that stretched over her sunken cheeks. Paper thin eyelids hung low over the cloudy gray orbs that floated deep in their sockets. I quickly looked away from this specter and sank to the floor, letting my back rest against the cool porcelain tub in anticipation of the next abdominal convulsion.

Someone knocked at the back entrance. Before I could move, the door unlatched; keys jingled in the lock. Footsteps followed through the kitchen. Seconds later, the bathroom door burst open, and my mother looked down at me across the threshold.

"We're going back to the hospital," she said, and I was in no condition to argue.

PART I

Out West or Anywhere

1

HE TOLD ME FROM THE BEGINNING he was going to move back out west. He had a dream to follow, and if he waited too long that dream would pass him by. This wasn't your usual, run-of-the-mill dream. Nick was going to be a dog musher. He'd spent the past two winters running sled dogs as a tour guide in Colorado. Before that he'd trained puppies for a couple of world-champion dog mushers in Alaska. But his real dream was to race, which meant having his own team in a place like Colorado or Idaho, where long winters produced enough snow to last the better part of most years. This pit stop at his father's house in central Pennsylvania was only temporary—a last-ditch fund-raising effort before taking the plunge to fulfill his destiny. Little did I know, as we sipped our salty margaritas on the night we first met, that Nick's destiny was like a creeping vine, thick and strong and already charting its path across the country. That vine reached across the table as we spoke, and my own unfledged destiny never saw it coming.

Drinks at Chi Chi's had been my coworker's idea which, bolstered by the restaurant's complementary chips and salsa policy, accommodated both my dinner budget and my general fondness for happy hour. Anne and I had worked together for almost two years, but this was our first social outing. Whether it had to do with our age difference or the fact that we worked different shifts didn't matter. I rarely turned down invitations where cocktails and food were involved. Sometime after the margarita order and before the arrival of our corn chip basket, her friend Nicolas showed up with a companion who looked to be about my age.

"I told Nicolas to bring his son," Anne said, as if I'd known Nicolas would be joining us. From the limited details she shared at work, it sounded as if she and Nicolas maintained an on-again, off-again, more-than-friend relationship that had spanned several decades. This kind of relationship I'd grown to regard as suspect after many years of living vicariously through my high school girlfriends who actually dated—an enterprise, at the age of twenty-six, I had yet to master.

"Nicky, this is Tara," said Anne, turning her attention to the younger of our surprise guests.

"Nicky?" I repeated before I could stop myself. He wore a black fleece vest over a plaid button-down shirt, and khaki cargo shorts that gave him the appearance of a Grand Canyon trail guide.

"It's Nick," he said, acknowledging the expanse of table between us and stuffing his hands into those cargo pockets.

"Nicky's staying with me for the summer," his father said, glancing in my direction by way, I presumed, of a greeting.

"That's nice," I offered, but he had already shifted his focus.

For the next forty-five minutes, I smiled and nodded and feigned general interest in the conversation, which centered around Corvettes and other such luxury cars—many of which Nicholas apparently owned. I finally gave up the act and turned my attention to the dwindling margarita in front of me, wishing the waiter would return with a double.

"Tara went to Australia for a semester," I heard Anne say, and I looked up from my glass, wiping the salt from my lips.

"Oh yeah?" Nick said. "When did you do that?"

"In college," I said, meeting his gaze. Nick's dark, wavy hair flopped over the sides of his head, and the rectangular, black-rimmed glasses he wore made me think of Buddy Holly. "I did an exchange my junior year."

"What was that like?" he asked, leaning across the table toward me. I looked into his steady brown eyes. They drooped, almost imperceptibly, at the rims, giving him a sad and world-wise countenance. Or that of a mischievous puppy, I imagined, depending on the circumstances.

"It was amazing," I said. "I took a seventeen-day bus tour of the Outback."

"Wow," he smiled broadly, revealing a gap between his two front teeth the width of a sideways Chiclet. "That sounds awesome."

"Nicky, do you remember that 650-horsepower vette?" his father broke in. "What was the sweet spot on that thing?"

"I don't know—," Nick glanced at the table and shrugged his shoulders, "what, about eighty?" he said and turned toward his father.

"It was eighty, wasn't it," his father laughed. Nick smiled again, and I thought of my mother. She had the same space between her two front teeth. I would have it too if she hadn't insisted on correcting it when I was eight years old.

Even with those imperfect teeth, Nick's smile was unguarded and confident—comfortable and familiar. *I could never be that way*, I thought, studying his features as my mind flashed back to the operation I'd had to fix my teeth. For months, I'd secured miniature rubber bands around those two front teeth in an effort to keep them from sliding back to their natural positions on opposite sides of my mouth.

"I just got back from Colorado." Nick turned his gaze on me, and I felt the color rise to my cheeks as I pulled my mind out of the memory. "I was working at a dog sled touring company," he said.

Before Colorado he had lived in Alaska. And before that, Arizona. This mop-headed car lover, I realized, was also an explorer. As I opened my mouth to ask what had attracted him to each of those places, Nick's father launched into a story about his helicopter. The conversation returned to the vehicles used for travel rather than the experiences gained in the process, and I held my tongue, having nothing of value to add.

When we said our goodbyes, Nick made his way to my side of the table and extended his hand. "It was very nice meeting you," he said, his hand warm and firm around mine. I looked up to meet his gaze. Then he smiled, gave my hand an extra squeeze, and turned to join his father at the door.

Though I'd freely admit that love at first sight was fine for people with certain personality types, like Snow White or Elizabeth Taylor, I'd never been a love-at-first-sight kind of a girl. Romance was not my specialty.

"Tara needs help with guys," a friend once said at a high school dance, loud enough for me to hear. Rather than solicit help, I chose to avoid the dating scene almost entirely. It wasn't until college that I realized I'd better amp up the motivation to find a boyfriend if I wanted to maintain the appearance of being a normal functioning human, which I definitely did. A friend fixed me up with a soccer player. Though the only thing we had in common may very well have been that friend, somehow, the relationship lasted for more than a year. When my boyfriend graduated and moved back to his hometown (and also immediately found someone else to date), he broke it off.

After college, I floundered with a few more attempts at romantic relationships, but it proved to be an area of weakness. By the age of twenty-six, I'd all but resigned myself to my future as a spinster-to-be. I might be running out of time to find a life partner, I thought, but there were plenty of years left to work on developing an affinity for cats.

It came as a shock when I arrived at work the week after we'd been to Chi-Chi's, and Anne told me that Nick had asked for my phone number.

"What could someone like Nick see in me?" I wondered out loud, switching on the computer at my station. As a graphic artist for a privately owned weather company, my job was to draw maps that would air on TV. It was a 24/7 operation, and I was on second shift. Anne had been there for three hours by the time I arrived and was clearly in no mood to converse. She shrugged, turned back to her drawing, and didn't broach the subject again until the end of her shift.

"So, what should I tell him?" she said as she stood to leave.

I took a deep breath and held it in for a moment. Then I turned to face her.

"He's only here for the summer, right?"

"That's what he says."

I'd already proven my incompetence in the serious relationship department. Perhaps I'd do better with a casual summer fling. In fact, I reasoned, taking the commitment out of the equation might just ease the pressure enough to allow me to have some fun.

"What could it hurt?" I said, finally.

The answer to that question would unfold, not by the end of the summer, but in the series of events I'd unknowingly triggered. Those events were now primed, like dominoes in a galactic maze, to topple one after another over the next four years of my life.

2

I WAS THREE YEARS OLD when my family moved to Lock Haven, Pennsylvania, where my father had secured a position as a music professor at Lock Haven State College. This was a significant upgrade from his previous position as a high school band teacher. The house my parents bought was affordable due to its location in a section of the Flemington borough that bore close proximity to several low-income housing developments and featured more than a few architectural eyesores (some so dilapidated my parents' house looked almost regal by comparison).

It was a red brick, two-story Colonial Revival built in 1938 on an acre of land—the ex-home, my parents would be reminded often, of the town's previous pharmacist. An elementary school sat on the opposite side of the street, though that would close before I reached the age to attend. We had three bedrooms—enough for my parents, my brother, and me, and one bath—enough only for me. It's possible my parents' choice to invest in the right house on the wrong side of town stemmed from my mother's deeply rooted dedication to pragmatism and fiscal restraint, which stemmed, in great part, from a childhood punctuated by periods of near destitution.

For me, the location fostered a developmental environment of full-tackle football and improvised games—all with my brother's friends—that involved hurling rocks at each other's heads while running for cover. Clearly, this neighborhood suffered from a double X chromosome drought. I tagged along with the boys for this reason and also because, shortly after I was born, my mother had bestowed my brother with the responsibility of my well-being in times of parental absence. Outside playtime always started with a warning. "She's your responsibility," my mother would say to Brian. He was sixteen months my senior.

Big events where I grew up were fistfights, and I'll never forget the first one I saw. All the neighborhood kids flocked to the playground behind the elementary school at the designated time of the fight. As the smallest member of the audience—one of only two girls in a sea of neighborhood boys—I stood at the back of the crowd, catching glimpses of the action in negative spaces between the shifting torsos and elbows in front of me. Rather than viewing the carnage, my interest lay solely in keeping up appearances as the rough-and-tumble tomboy I believed myself to be. For the first time, I heard the sound of fist on flesh and thought I saw a spattering of blood. The nausea that followed was new and palpable. But it didn't deter me from believing I was as tough as any boy. Growing up in my neighborhood was enough to convince me of that.

Maybe the reason I ached so badly for a pet, most painfully a puppy, in those years had something to do with my inability to fit in or find compatible playmates, given those neighborhood dynamics. But persistent pleading in the pet department proved no match for my mother's resolve.

"Animals are dirty," she would say when I brought up the subject, as if it were a reasonable excuse. She had been known to refer to herself as "house proud" and was disinclined to share her house with a bunch of dirty, smelly animals.

Her sister, Aunt Janet, had kept an eclectic mix of pets in the house when they were children. She'd save the live "peeps" they received as Easter presents each year, their feathery chick fuzz dyed pink, green, or blue, and she'd raise them in a home-made chicken coop right in the bedroom that she and my mother shared. "I'll never forget that smell," my mother said to me more than once.

I suppose those childhood circumstances contributed to her aversion to indoor animals, though this realization came long after it mattered. I begged for a pet all the single-digit years of my life, and what I got instead were sterile equivalents—a stuffed basset hound named Baxter with a head so large it toppled him over; a miniature chestnut pony with a white blaze and a straw-colored mane, permanently lying on its side; and an Afghan hound with an acrylic blonde coat, featured with my arms encircling its stiff neck in the family Christmas photo snapped the morning Santa had left it under our tree.

I appeased my yearning for four-legged companionship by befriending all the stray animals I could find in our neighborhood. I'd win the occasional goldfish at a carnival when I was really trying for the cuddly bunny or the fuzzy duckling you'd win if you landed your plastic ping-pong ball in the smallest fishbowl at the top of the fishbowl pyramid. Fish weren't cuddly, though, and mine never lasted long.

"I'm not going to have babies when I grow up," I informed my mother every so often. "I'm going to have puppies!"

It wasn't until I'd reached junior high, and my longing for a puppy had faded, that we finally got one. We'd gone as a family to a dog show, and the shelties had impressed my father. I'll never know how he convinced my mother to allow such a hairy breed into the house. I did discover that our new puppy wasn't solely for the children. My dad had a master plan. He wanted to compete with the sheltie, and he groomed that dog for at least an hour every day to cultivate his future champion. Dad's expectations always did exceed perfection (an influence so ingrained in me, I wouldn't know to refute it until it was almost too late). But the dog dropped only one testicle. My father had gotten him at half price with the breeder saying the second testicle was likely to drop.

Our sheltie never did win in the ring, and he wasn't what I'd had in mind as a little girl looking for a partner in adolescence—an object for my homeless affection. By ninth grade, a scab-like crust had formed around the tender core of my previously exposed feelings, and by the time I left for college, that scab had hardened, almost imperceptibly and of its own volition, into a thick layer of impenetrable scar tissue.

Shortly after leaving for college, I went home for a family cookout. I opened the kitchen cupboard to find a glass and spotted something familiar, high on an unreachable shelf. It was the mug I'd made for my mother as a Valentine's Day present in second grade, a precursor to today's customized porcelain mugs with the photographs of children or grandchildren or beloved dogs screened seamlessly on. My mug was made of milky white plastic and featured a clear plastic face behind which I'd inserted my Valentine's message. I'd trimmed a sheet of white construction paper to the specifications necessary to fit neatly around the perimeter of the mug. Onto that paper I'd pasted my second-grade photo—my mother's favorite—then used a red magic marker to fill the paper with vibrant hearts of all shapes and sizes. Above the photo of the freckle-faced girl with the long brown pigtails who struggled to smile, as her mother had begged her to do in spite of the embarrassment of missing her two front teeth, appeared the words, "I love you!"

I wondered when that mug had been relegated to the untouchable shelf with the fine china and still-in-the-box Waterford crystal. I also wondered, as I extracted my glass and closed the cupboard door that afternoon, if the mug I'd crafted as a second-grade art project represented the last time I'd ever said "I love you" to my mother.

3

I TOOK EXTREME MEASURES to escape the male-dominated confines of Flemington, staying with girlfriends I'd met in school as often as possible. A few families may as well have adopted me based on the amount of time I spent in their homes, not to mention the extra money they must have shelled out in grocery bills on my behalf. Where the cupboards in my house might offer up a can of tuna fish and a half a tube of Unsalted Tops saltine crackers in a hunger pinch, my friends' homes featured pantries stocked with potato chips, cookies, TastyKakes, conveniently boxed rice and pasta meals—even sugary cereals as opposed to the Raisin Bran, Corn Flakes, or Cheerios occupying the otherwise barren cupboards in my home. One family went so far as to designate their guest room as "Tara's bedroom" after years of my persistent presence.

But the neighborhood wasn't the only contributing factor to my home life avoidance. In close quarters, my mother and I created an unbalanced electromagnetic field that proved anti-conducive to co-existence. My father and brother contributed to the supercharged atmosphere with their own unstable personality elements. Explosions in this environment occurred frequently and without warning. On rare Saturday mornings at home, I often awoke to the nerve-shredding alarm of my parents' shouting matches.

When on the verge of a rage, my mother's tension spread through the house like the waft of charged air before an electrical storm. I sensed her moods more keenly than my brother, who tormented me in a creative variety of ways, regardless of her nerves. Sometimes, he would pin me down on the living room carpet and dribble a gob of phlegm millimeters above my face before sucking it back into his mouth. Often he would tickle me until tears streamed from my eyes and I could no longer breathe. Always, he would practice the moves he'd learned watching WWF (then the World Wrestling Federation) on TV.

I was a screamer. I screamed for mercy and I screamed for help and eventually, inevitably, my screams awoke the beast. My mother often napped during the day when Brian and I were young. If my screams woke her up, she'd fly down the stairs in a rage after both of us. Spanking was the norm back then, and my brother and I both got our share.

Brian took the brunt of the punishment, especially from my father, who successfully bottled his rage for longer periods of time. Where my mother's temper came in short, frequent bursts, my father's anger flared like lightning, and the residual thunder rumbled after. I felt the force of my father's temper once. Something I'd said or done provoked his anger, and I tripped as he chased me up the stairs; or perhaps he caught my ankle. Either way, I'll never forget the venom in his eyes as he hovered over me with a ready fist, the breath from his clenched jaw coming in hot, short bursts against my face. His lips curled back to expose sharp, grinding teeth. Those teeth were known to sever fishing line. He never hit me. He didn't have to. I was the sensitive one who learned through fear.

Over the years, I grew quiet. My mother would call me "the only Indian in a family of chiefs," which I interpreted to mean she thought I was a follower rather than a leader. I didn't feel like a follower, but I did learn to act like one. And if you act a certain way long enough, you are certain to assimilate the qualities you've been pretending to possess.

I'd entertain myself for hours on end, drawing or writing stories or making art projects with the piles of multi-colored construction paper, crayons, and scissors we kept under the living room couch. At one point, I believed I could fly. I'd done it before, I insisted to my mother. All I had to do was stand at the top of the stairs and spin a certain way to levitate a few inches in the air. Then I'd slowly twirl my way down the stairs to the landing.

This may have been what I was attempting after my bath one evening when I stood wrapped in a towel at the top of the thirteen-step staircase. The next thing I knew I was tumbling, and by the time I reached the landing, my father was there to catch me. He'd been taking a nap in the TV room. The second he heard me falling, he leapt from his chair and sprinted through the living room to the bottom of the stairs. I looked up from his arms as he pushed the sleeping blinders from his eyes—he'd run the whole way without seeing. What I saw in his eyes was raw terror at the thought that his child might be injured. My father, I knew then, would do anything to protect me.

The dichotomy between my parents' deep love for my brother and me and their volatile tempers confused me. I never knew when my brother would pounce or when my mother would unleash her rage. Any step

I took in my own home might detonate a land mine for which I had no defense. I developed skin rashes, canker sores, and eye twitches. I complained almost daily of stomachaches.

"Is she an overachiever?" the doctor asked when my mother questioned him about my maladies. Upon hearing that I was, he informed her that we overachievers were well-known complainers. It was normal for me to say my tummy hurt when I ate Hillbilly wheat bread. "Best to ignore it," he assured her.

I would later learn that my stomach problems started when I was nine months old. I'd had diarrhea for weeks. At the doctor's recommendation, my mother put me on what she called a "starvation diet." I once saw a photograph of me taken during that time. The baby in the photo had an ethereal presence, like a porcelain doll with ocean blue glass eyes—a doll that might break if you touched it. After a full week on nothing but Pedialyte, my health had not improved. When the same doctor informed my mother she was now starving me, she plunged with characteristic resolution into a tactic that bordered on force-feeding. Her sheer will restored me to good health and an even healthier baby weight within weeks.

The stomachaches continued through adolescence. I would lie in bed at night, looking up at the ceiling where my dragon friend, cast by the shadows thrown by the nightlight, watched over me. "I'm going to die of stomach cancer," I predicted, holding my protruding potbelly as I said it. I couldn't have been more than six years old at the time.

Not all of my maladies could be written off as imaginary. My first cavity appeared when I was in second grade. I jumped out of the chair and into my dad's arms, initially refusing to allow the dentist (who also happened to be my uncle) to fill the defective tooth. In addition to a few more cavities that required filling over the years after that first encounter, I developed other enamel abnormalities that couldn't be explained, including a variety of discolorations and soft spots. For the remainder of my childhood, I lived in fear that any one of those soft spots would decay into a full-blown cavity that would require invasive and painful eradication the next time I went in for a routine cleaning.

Such was the nature of anxiety, an affliction that had plagued the maternal side of my family for generations. My mother suffered. My grammie suffered. And Grammie's mother suffered before that. My stomachaches were inevitable, I came to conclude, as the unique way our family's genetic anxiety manifested in me.

The only person I confided in was Grammie, the single stable element of my post-pubescent youth. When trouble brewed at home, Grammie's apartment was my escape. Regardless of which action had pushed my mother to the razor's edge of sanity, prompting her recurring threat to "beat me to a bloody pulp," unconditional love awaited me at Grammie's. I "ran away from home" to Grammie's apartment on a semi-regular basis. My longest stay was a week.

Grammie's apartment felt like home in a way my real home did not. It smelled like meatloaf in the oven and fresh Pepperidge Farm toast. Warm things. Comfort and love. She offered up her best chair every time I visited—a plush La-Z-Boy recliner the likes of which my mother would never allow in her home because, as she repeated each time my father expressed interest in purchasing one for the TV room, reclining chairs were "ugly."

In Grammie's reclining chair, I found beautiful solace. I'd curl up in that cushy La-Z-Boy with Grammie's miniature schnauzer beside me, her warm body thawing my heart. I'd sometimes show up in tears, having recruited my brother to drive me the ten miles to Grammie's apartment because I didn't have a car of my own. By that time our quarreling had run its course, and we'd grown to feel more like allies than enemies. If our home was a war zone, the least my brother and I could do was acknowledge our solidarity in the matter.

Grammie always kept food in the house for my impromptu visits. Comfort food she could make into a meal or junk food, like cheese puffs, I could snack on all night long. Sometimes I'd binge until my stomach ached, then Grammie would offer me a cup of hot peppermint water to soothe my tummy. At some point in the evening, the phone would ring, and Grammie's muffled voice would drift to where I was sitting in the next room. "She's safe," I'd hear her say, and something inside me would settle in the knowledge that my parents had checked.

At least once a year and sometimes twice throughout senior high, Grammie and I embarked on what became known as one of our signature shopping sprees. We'd lap the mall twice—the first time to scope out the clothes that caught my eye and the second to narrow down the selection to articles deemed purchase-worthy after multiple trips to the fitting room. We'd return to a store a third time if I still couldn't make up my mind, which happened more frequently than not. Grammie would have to find a chair by the second lap, but she never once suggested we cut our shopping short. She may have fought off a diabetic low-blood-sugar attack in the midst of it all, but she did not lose patience with me during those extended shopping extravaganzas.

After satiating my appetite for apparel, Grammie would take me to the restaurant of my choice, and I'd order an ice cream sundae for dinner while she struggled to get her sugar levels back on track.

At her apartment, I'd conduct a fashion show of the outfits we'd bought that day, taking care to demonstrate all the ways the Benetton sweaters and Esprit button-down shirts (or as Grammie called them, blouses) mixed and matched with my Guess jeans and Liz Claiborne pants (otherwise known as slacks). Sometimes Grammie would take pictures, and we'd always end up in a fit of hysterical laughter when one of us remembered the speed and proficiency with which she had devoured her pudding cup or whatever typically forbidden treat she'd consumed to get her sugar levels back under control earlier in the day.

"Tell me a story," I'd coax when I got into bed, though I was much too old for bedtime stories.

"Oh, I've told you all my stories," she'd say, and I'd beg her until she gave in. She'd share a childhood memory involving long-lost cousins or her brother before he was killed conducting a routine flight at the end of WWII. I'd fall asleep with the fairy dust of Grammie's nostalgia fluttering through my dreams, leaving behind a tinge of sadness in its wake.

My mother avoided shopping and anything involving thick crowds (such was the unique manifestation of her genetic anxiety). And she either would not or could not spend the kind of money it would take for me to dress like my friends. If it hadn't been for Grammie and those shopping sprees, I'd have entered high school clad in my grade-school wardrobe, which consisted of Wrangler's carpenter jeans and too-small T-shirts typically featuring a company logo, like LEE™, on the chest. The problem was, the friends I'd made in elementary school had risen to the ranks of wardrobe judges in junior high. If I wanted to keep those friends, and I saw no other option, it was clear I would have to share their interests. Clothing was just the beginning.

I joined the cheerleading squad, abandoned the artistic inclinations of my youth, and eventually started going to keg parties. I stopped speaking to my parents and passed the time at home in my bedroom with the door closed. I listened to music. I talked on the phone. I scribbled in my journal—clumsy poems, pregnant with angst and carelessly aborted. Even that made me feel too exposed. By senior high, I recoiled from my journal as well.

My father resorted to lectures, corralling me into the sun room (also known as the music room) and pacing while he shuffled through his 3" x 5" index cards for terms like "dangerous path" and "on the ledge." I sat on the piano bench and glared unblinking at a discolored splotch in the floorboard. His efforts only stoked my fury. I wondered if he used similar index cards with the students in his courses.

I allowed my parents access into my teenage life only when they offered me something, like a trip to Dairy Queen or a ride to meet up with friends. My grades dropped without fanfare, and by senior year, I gave all appearance of fitting the demographic addressed by the principal in his speech to our graduating class. "Ninety five percent of you in this room are going to fail," he told us, and I knew enough to tune the rest of his words out.

I had been smart once, I vaguely remembered. I would prove that I could be again, as soon as I escaped the suffocating clutches of high school. In the meantime, I walked the locker-lined halls with a sour face and a morose outlook, which my friends somehow came to accept as part of my natural personality.

One of those friends would pick me up every Friday and Saturday night. She'd sit outside my parents' house in her Yugo or her Pinto or her Ford Fiesta, beeping the horn every ten minutes or so in an effort to inspire me to hurry. But hurry was not in my vocabulary. Along with refining my fashion, I'd learned to apply makeup and style my hair. These enhancements took time for a recovering tomboy like myself. So my friends would wait, upward of an hour, while I finished perfecting my eyeliner or positioning each strand of my hair. And my family would wait, not always in good humor, for access to our home's only bathroom.

My costumes only went so far. Underneath the makeup and designer clothes lived a naked insecurity, a crushing self-consciousness born of a sensitive and scared little girl—a girl who'd had a lot of love to give at one point in her life. A girl whose love, over many years, had folded tightly in on itself. What used to be love now sat like a stone in my heart.

While my friends all paired off with boys, I kept to myself, or I hung out with whichever girlfriend happened to be dateless on any given evening. I grew into the role of listener and adviser—the one who was always there when you needed her. My friends bestowed me with labels like "grounded" and "down to earth." They came to me for an "honest opinion." This did not always work in my favor. Sometimes a friend would ignore me for weeks after receiving the "honest opinion" she had sought. Refraining from dating afforded me the luxury of relying on theory-based opinions. I not so silently judged my friends for compromising their values and, per my point of view, losing themselves in their romantic relationships.

"You don't know what you're missing," a friend said to me once. But I felt justified in maintaining my safe distance and reliable perspective each time such a friend approached me with a new relationship dilemma.

I knew all the boys wanted my prettier, more popular friends. I was just the tagalong—the girl someone might go out with if her better-looking friend was not available. I convinced myself that any boy who acted interested was merely settling and, therefore, did not deserve me. I lopped off romantic advances with expert precision. All I typically had to do was stand back long enough for another girl to swoop in and divert the boy's attention. If that failed, I tried avoidance. If he persisted, I went for the jugular with a straightforward rejection.

Once, at a weekend dance held in the high school gymnasium, a boy asked me to slow dance with him. I considered us friends, though he'd hinted at having interest in more. While we danced, he confided that he sometimes thought about suicide. "That's selfish," I said, abolishing the subject entirely. We finished our dance in silence, and our friendship faded shortly thereafter. By that time in my life, I knew how to keep my emotional distance. And I did it without mercy.

4

THE PRIMARY GOAL when I thought about college involved living far away from my hometown. Though my parents said it wasn't an option, I knew that anything was possible. I did not, on the other hand, know about student loans, grants, or other financial aid opportunities. My performance in high school voided the possibility of a scholarship. Tuition would be free where my father taught, and the college had been upgraded to a university in the Pennsylvania State System of Higher Education since he began his career there.

It wasn't my first choice, but I had no clue as to how to arrive at a first choice. The only skill I'd acquired in high school was that of navigating the educational system without actually learning anything. No teacher or guidance counselor talked to me about my areas of strength, let alone helped me to choose a school based on them. My parents, by that time, were too far removed from my personal life to point me in a purposeful direction. For all anyone knew, including myself as a high-school graduate, I no longer had any areas of strength.

I chose journalism as a major because writing was the only skill I'd at one time possessed that I thought I might be able to resurrect. (Though my mother would point out, when I signed up to be the features co-editor of the student-run newspaper the following year, that I'd never read a newspaper in my life.) Prior to agreeing to attend the university of my parents' choice, I bargained with them for a foreign exchange trip. I'd read about Lock Haven University's study abroad program in the recruitment brochures I'd received in the mail. If my parents would pay for me to study in Australia for a semester, I supposed I could put my long-term escape plans on hold for a few more years. Not only did they agree to the semester abroad, they offered to pay for my room and board on campus starting immediately. My parents were just as anxious to get me out of their house as I was to escape.

I headed to the dorms that summer. Almost immediately, the autonomy of living away from home, or the flexibility of a college schedule, or the natural hormone changes of adulthood, or some magic combination thereof melted my teenaged angst into a more fluid substance—one that navigated in harmony with, rather than clashing and colliding against the environment it inhabited.

My father invited me to concerts, and I soon found that I shared his interest in music. He would treat me to dinner at a fancy restaurant before taking me to a Yo-Yo Ma or a Maynard Ferguson concert. Then he'd talk about the music or the musician from his perspective as a music professor with no 3" x 5" index cards in sight.

Around that time, my mother introduced me to independent and foreign films. We'd sip chardonnay and spend entire afternoons watching movies and nibbling on French bread dipped in cheese fondue. I would later name a car after a film we'd watched on such an afternoon. Betty Blue, my car would be called. She would one day carry me farther away from my family than I could have imagined on the afternoon my mother and I sipped our wine and watched the original Betty gouge out her eye with a spoon.

I was sure my parents still fought like an alley cat and a Jack Russell terrier, but spending time with them separately kept me from having to witness it. I refused to subject myself to the battlegrounds of my past by spending unnecessary time at home. My mother must have intuited this message. She changed the dynamic, at least on special occasions, by introducing the holiday jug of wine. Getting together for holidays had always been a priority in my family, but the addition of wine to our gatherings created a different emotional dimension entirely. Something about combining an extravagant home-cooked meal with copious amounts of Chianti made my parents lighten up enough to get through the day without major combat. The jug effectively quelled my mother's instinct to scream at my father when he set the wrong silverware for the holiday meal. And the day I heard my father *ask* which silverware to set, I knew a principle element of their relationship had shifted, if only on these isolated occasions.

With the jug on the table, our conversations went from virtually nonexistent to borderline jovial. We discussed everything from philosophical concepts to childhood memories, my brother and I laughing to the verge of hysterics at the recollection of sprinting through the house in terror-stricken circles—through the living room and into the TV room and through the kitchen then down the hallway and back into the living room and through the TV room and into the kitchen— followed closely by our enraged mother and the dreaded wooden spoon she wielded that would do who knew what extent of damage if it ever connected.

"What did we do to deserve it that time?" my brother would ask as we sat at the dinner table, and I would raise my hand to be called on for a response.

"I think it might have been the time you saw Jimmy Superfly Snuka on TV and felt the need to practice the super flying body splash on me by jumping off the dining room chair." It was the same every time.

"Oh yeah," my brother would laugh, "and you screamed bloody murder until Mom got out of bed and pounded down the stairs to get the wooden spoon!"

The conversation would continue with Dad shaking his head in what I interpreted as disbelief. I often wondered if his disbelief stemmed from the events that had transpired at home while he worked at the university all day or from the fact that we now laughed about them. Mom would sometimes offer a self-defensive qualifier like "They said sibling rivalry was normal back then," and my brother and I would laugh even harder.

Those bolstered conversations kept us coming back to the family hub for good holiday times several times a year. The jug became a tradition until the jug was no longer *en vogue* and we classed it up by moving to smaller, two-liter bottles.

I spent the first semester of my junior year in Australia where, between near-constant traveling and perpetual partying, I somehow completed an internship at a biweekly newspaper. I considered studying in Spain during my senior year, but fate, I soon learned, had different plans for me. I was using the ATM at the edge of campus one afternoon the semester after I returned from Australia when the man in line behind me offered his congratulations. I searched his face for a clue of recognition.

"I'm Bill," he said. "We haven't met. I'm a news reporter for the *Eagle Eye* now, and I've read your work." The *Eagle Eye* was the university's student-run, weekly newspaper. I'd been co-editor of the features section prior to going abroad.

"Ah," I said, awaiting further details.

"Haven't you heard? You're the new editor-in-chief."

"Really?" I hadn't known I was in the running. "Thanks," I said. "And no, I hadn't heard."

I assumed my advisor had nominated me for the position, though I never did confirm the suspicion. Whatever had transpired, it seemed ungrateful to turn down an opportunity practically handed to me on a silver platter. I accepted the position, which would start that summer and run through my senior year.

In the twelve months that followed, I worked harder than I'd ever worked in my life, often sleeping less than ten hours from Monday through Friday as I tackled my course load and ran the paper. I'd write my editorial on the morning of publication day, spending the night in the office after everyone had left. Around 6:00 a.m., I'd finish pasting up the paper and run the galleys to the local newspaper's press in time to make the 7:00 a.m. deadline for printing. Then I'd stop at my apartment for a shower and walk the mile back to campus for my 8:00 a.m. class.

That first semester as editor-in-chief, I lost ten pounds, and those strange maladies from childhood crept back into my life. In the shower one morning, I noticed several hard lumps in my groin area. My mind leapt immediately to the worst-case scenario, which seemed most likely to be malignant tumors. I knew I had to find a doctor ASAP. I chose one I'd known as a young child when his wife and my mother were friends. I'd grown up with this doctor's children, which I thought might reduce the humiliation of requesting a groin examination. It did not, and neither did the doctor's final diagnosis of swollen glands. To be thorough or empathetic, he ordered blood work, the results of which prompted a prescription for iron supplements. My anemia would prove chronic and severe.

"You really should have a blood transfusion," he told me after the iron supplements he'd prescribed triggered the same vein of intestinal distress and bowel purging I'd battled as a child. I acknowledged his suggestion as absurd. Instead of forcing the issue, this family friend found an iron supplement touted as being easier on the digestive system. But those supplements made me feel worse than the first. Rather than risk another threat of transfusion, I threw the pills in the garbage and never contacted that doctor again.

I'd read somewhere—perhaps in my roommate's copy of Cosmo—that most women my age were anemic. Clearly, it was possible to live with this condition.

The resulting burnout from serving as editor-in-chief compelled me to abandon any notions of becoming a career journalist. Instead, I remained in school for an extra year to complete a dual major in psychology. I folded my writing education neatly up with my experience and stuffed the package into my back pocket. It would be a hobby, I thought—a skill I could summon, in the way I might whip out my driver's license when I needed it. "Writing is something you can do anywhere," people often said, and it made sense. My new plan involved finding freedom and independence out west.

I applied to graduate programs for clinical psychology in Colorado and Oregon, but none of my applications were accepted. So I settled into a part-time job in my hometown, caring for residents with cognitive disabilities in a group home. When I heard that two girls I'd known in high school were planning to drive across the country and spend a month exploring before looking for jobs at a ski resort, I knew my chance had come. They planned to camp along the way to keep expenses low. My contributions, I pointed out, would further reduce their travel costs.

I'd saved enough money to last for a month and, though I wasn't much of a skier, I figured any job I found would pay better than the four dollars and meager change I was making per hour at the group home. I would have to fly back to Pennsylvania for my best friend's wedding in mid-October, but it was only September. We'd have at least three weeks to explore before that. After the wedding, I'd rejoin my friends out west to look for an apartment and find a job for the winter.

I gave notice to leave my position at the end of summer. Then off we went, motoring across the country to see the Badlands and Mount Rushmore, Yellowstone and Old Faithful, Las Vegas and Death Valley, and finally, the Grand Canyon. It was the tail end of September, and we were camping in the desert. For three nights at the Canyon, my friends and I cuddled in our sleeping bags like pack dogs, sharing body warmth. We stayed a fourth day to go on the classic western wagon ride and weenie roast we'd signed up for when we arrived. The decision to leave directly after was unanimous.

I sat hunched in the back seat of my friend's pine green Subaru sedan as we sped toward the Four Corners border. Those weenies had not settled in my stomach. It was ten o'clock at night when we pulled into the parking lot of a convenience store in a dusty town we later learned was part of the Navajo Nation. Kayenta, the sign read. It looked like a ghost town to us.

I saw the dog from the corner of my eye as I exited the car—an orange ball of fur curled up like a fox on the mat outside the door I'd have to walk through to retrieve the bathroom key. I'd seen so many strays by that point in our travels I'd adopted an emotional defense mechanism. I stared straight ahead, knowing that a split-second glance would launch my heart in the same direction and, while my eyes would inevitably return to their forward-facing focus, the heart was more likely to stick, indefinitely, to the fuzzy orange target.

I made a clear first and second pass, barely noticing the wide eyes that followed my every movement. The rest of the dog's face was hidden, tucked under its plume of a tail. Leaving the bathroom, I braced myself for the third pass, but the dog did not appear in my peripheral vision. I looked directly at the mat. It was vacant. *Lucky*, I thought, glancing toward the car where I now saw my companions, fawning all over the emaciated canine.

I returned the key then crouched to stroke the feathery red fur framing the scrawny dog's face. Its pointed ears were almost as big as its head. As I stood to open the car door, the fox-dog exerted all the effort it must have had in that malnourished body to lift itself up on hind legs and extend its two front paws slowly upward as far as they could stretch. Soft brown eyes gazed into mine with what I could only interpret as hope. "Up?" the dog seemed to say in the same way a small child might ask when her fledgling legs fail to carry her. That's when my heart launched and stuck.

The fox-dog chased us as we drove away, sprinting down the darkened road after the car. My friend thought the dog might belong to the person working in the convenience store—a logical conclusion that set my mind at ease. We agreed to return and ask the clerk to keep it inside while we drove away. Traveling slowly in the dim light of a slivered moon, we noted, with collective curiosity, a surprising number of leashless and unescorted dogs materializing as shadows and disappearing beyond the edge of darkness.

"Did you see that?" we questioned, unsure of the validity of our visions. After several moments, enough of these ghost dogs appeared to prompt a stop at a gas station where a police officer stood, filling up the tank of his patrol car.

"Strays," the officer said when we asked him about the shadow dogs. "The pound comes on Tuesdays to round them up, so if you see one you like, you might as well take it."

We drove in silence back to the convenience store, and the fox-dog reappeared in the parking lot. Rather than invite it in, the clerk confirmed that the dog was a stray. An ensuing discussion in the parking lot ended with my friends granting me the deciding vote on how to deal with the newest turn of events. I looked down at the dog, who gazed back at me with those wide-eyes, and I cast my ballot by opening the car door for the little fox-dog to jump in. We discovered that our new friend was female and named her Katy as we drove into the night toward Colorado.

When I returned to Pennsylvania for the wedding, I found a single message blinking on my answering machine. It was an invitation to interview for my first full-time job—the graphic artist position I would accept at the weather company in State College, less than forty miles from my hometown.

My travel companions moved on to Utah, where they found their ski-resort jobs. They searched for weeks to find a rental unit that allowed dogs before calling to tell me it was hopeless.

"I'll take her," I said without hesitating.

What I'd suspected when I agreed to the interview had now been confirmed. I would not be rejoining my friends out west. Instead, I borrowed money from Grammie to pay for Katy's plane ticket. Then I asked or, rather, informed my parents they would have to drive me to the Philadelphia airport—200 miles each way—to help me collect my new stray reservation dog. Perhaps they doubted the soundness of my decision to adopt a dog when I had no stable source of income and lived, at the time, in a pet-unfriendly apartment. But they drove me to the airport without argument.

As far as abandoning the original plan to live out west and share the rent with my travel companions, I assuaged the majority of my guilt through finely tuned powers of rationalization. I had cast the deciding vote to keep Katy, which rendered me responsible for her well-being. The moment I opened the car door and coaxed her to jump in that night on the Indian reservation, I knew that Katy was my dog. This was the companion I'd longed for since I was a little girl. Taking responsibility for Katy would solidify my independence. It was time to grow up, and the way to do that was by settling down and providing a stable home for my dog.

Two weeks later, I started my first full-time job. The path to my future had unfolded, and Pennsylvania was where I would stay. It had worked out for the best, considering I was not the least bit interested in living in Utah.

5

I MET NICK shortly after a brief affair (and inevitable breakup) with a meteorologist. This weatherman was smart and good-natured, and more than one person likened his looks to JFK Junior's. Not even six months into dating, he "met someone else." It occurred to me that the situation with my college boyfriend had been similar. And I'd had the same experience with one other person after that. This third time, I recognized a pattern that abolished all previous doubt; I was truly unlovable.

When Nick asked for my phone number, my inclination was to run. Somewhere along the line of my life, I had missed the lesson on how to participate in a functional romantic relationship, and I wasn't likely to learn at this stage. My primary long-term relationship was now with my dog who, I knew, would not abandon me for someone she liked better. Satisfaction as a single person hovered within my grasp, whereas embarking on another doomed relationship was more likely to shatter my hard-earned and newly acquired peace.

But something about Nick—this wiry adventurer who was taut with potential energy and different than anyone I'd ever known—intrigued me. He stood about five foot six and weighed close to 145 pounds. A set of unusually broad shoulders required him to wear extra-large tops, and the tops he chose typically consisted of flannel or fleece—fashions that made him look environmentally conscious but not redneck. I found his broad shoulders attractive and wondered if this had something to do with my affinity for mountain gorillas, gleaned over years of paging through my father's supply of National Geographic magazines.

More often than not, Nick's flannel or fleece featured creative yet functional designs like water-wicking insulation or armpit ventilating flaps. Such features fascinated me on a multitude of levels. For one, I hadn't known they existed. Even more enchanting was the revelation that a member of the opposite sex would take such meticulous interest in the design of his everyday clothing. I'd grown up around flannel-wearing boys. The kind who also wore baseball caps and construction boots and Levi's jeans, featuring a tell-tale ring in at least one of the back pockets. I'd never thought of those boys as people who would care to ventilate their armpits, nor did I consider their flannel fashions to be anything but ordinary. Nick's variety of multi-functional flannel made him seem both smart *and* sensitive. It was the sensitivity that hooked me.

He'd graduated from Boston University with a bachelor's degree having something to do with environmental studies. I had no idea if environmental studies had been available at Lock Haven University, but I certainly didn't know anyone who'd pursued it. It seemed a worthy cause in a world where people cared mostly about money and materials. Nick was different, I could tell already. After college, he had moved to Arizona to work for the Tribal Game and Fish Department at an Indian reservation. That's where he'd found his dog. Apparently, he bartered the puppy away from a Native American girl. As long as he named the dog after an Apache leader, the girl's grandfather had stipulated, he was welcome to take it. Chief Cochise it was (though most often shortened to Chief)—a now eighty-pound mix with the thick white coat of a malamute, the hanging ears of a Lab that perked smartly at the sound of anything resembling food or prey, and the look of the wild in his black-rimmed, amber eyes. Katy adored Chief. Chief regarded Katy in the same way an adolescent boy might tolerate his pesky younger sister.

Nick took his affinity for dogs and appreciation of the natural world, as he did most of his interests, to extremes—a captivating quality evidenced by his work on the Indian reservation and with sled dog racing. Nothing I'd worked toward in my life felt as meaningful as the things Nick had already accomplished with his. Like me, he had planned to go to graduate school. He'd been accepted in California but had dropped out when he couldn't find a place to live with his dog. Constant companions since their first meeting in Arizona, Nick and Chief were a traveling duo—two bachelors going wherever they pleased whenever it suited them until the summer of 1997 when they returned to central Pennsylvania for a visit. That visit, against all plans to the contrary, would extend through the better part of two years.

On the night we met at Chi-Chi's, Nick's hair was long and fuzzy and skirting the borderline of control. When he laughed, he clapped his hands together and threw his head back with disarming abandon, openly revealing the sizable gap between his two front teeth. Twenty years after I'd had the operation to eliminate the space between my own teeth, Nick would inform me some African cultures considered that gap to be sexy. He was always sharing randomly useful or thought-provoking wisdom nuggets. I didn't know about sexy, but I had to admit, that gap did endear Nick to me.

He once said that two people in a relationship should naturally make each other better people. Profound words to live by, I thought. He told me it wasn't normal to have all the stomachaches I had. Of course, I knew it was normal for me.

Shortly after we started seeing each other, I returned home from work to find a two-liter Coke bottle cut off at the top and filled with vibrant wildflowers on the doorstep. *How creative*, I thought, as I carried them into the house. Later that evening, Nick stopped by unannounced. When I thanked him for the flowers, he said he wanted to be clear.

"About what?" I asked.

"I want to be more than friends," he said. And then he kissed me.

From that time on, vases in various forms—whatever Nick could find in his car when the picking mood struck—showed up on my doorstep brimming with wildflowers of yellow and white and multiple shades of purple. Every bouquet was different, and the novelty of those spontaneous arrangements never wore off.

Nick opened doors and pulled out chairs and even refrained from speeding past cars on two-lane roads when we were together. "Not with the pretty girl in the car," he would say, reaching over with his shifting hand to give my knee a squeeze.

Up to that point, I'd maintained what I thought was a progressive outlook on the male to female dynamic. I held no qualms about opening doors for men or pulling out my own chair, but something about Nick's old-school manners made me doubt my unlovable status. The tinge of guilt that struck every time I waited for Nick to open the passenger-side car door inspired me to question my stance on gender equality.

My boyfriend called me names like "pretty girl" and "sweetie"—terms outside of my comfort zone and therefore off limits before Nick came along. The hypocrisy I noted in myself did not preclude me from basking in the treatment. This newfound femininity felt like something worth exploring, if not quite yet the perfect fit.

Things we enjoyed doing together included trying new restaurants—especially new dishes at new restaurants, taking our dogs for walks in the woods, and traveling. Things that only Nick enjoyed but that we did together anyway included fishing, clearing brush away from tree stands to prepare for hunting season, and openly talking about our feelings.

About a month after we met, he took me to a cabin that a friend of his father owned. The property was gated, and we picked up the key on the way to the cabin where we planned to spend the night. Nick had brought his fishing rod, and, from the pond in front of the cabin, he planned to catch our dinner.

We set the dogs free to roam the property then opened a couple of beers and sat on the dock, holding hands and gazing at the horizon beyond the water. The day was hot and still. Nick pulled out his fishing rod as the sun descended toward the distant mountains. His line and sinker cast a soft ripple through the scattered clouds reflected in the pond's glassy surface. I sat cross-legged beside Nick as our dogs lay panting behind us on the dock. I glanced back at Katy. Her eyes squinted against the sun as she gazed across the pond, and her mouth gaped open in the shape of a smile.

The fishing line jerked, and Nick yanked his pole back to set the hook.

"Got one," he said, slowly reeling in the catch.

By the time he caught another, both of our stomachs were rumbling, and we decided two seven-inch brown trout would suffice for our dinner. Nick gathered some wood and kindling for the fire then squirted some lighter fluid onto the wood to speed its ignition. He gutted and cleaned the fish before dredging the filets in flour. Then he tossed the coated fish in an oil-treated, cast iron skillet he had brought for the occasion. The fresh filets sizzled in the heat of the fire, and I closed my eyes, the scent of the mingling oils wafting around me. We ate with our fingers as the trout cooled in the pan because we'd forgotten to bring any utensils.

Before dusk turned to dark, we pulled our sleeping bags out of Nick's Jeep and laid them on the mattress we'd found on the floor inside the cabin.

"I guess it's better than a tent," I said without thinking. Nick touched my face in the now fading light, and I looked up at him, suddenly nervous. He leaned in to kiss my lips. I let my tongue slip against his, softly at first, and then deeper as I relaxed into his arms. His hands caressed the small of my back, gently urging. A tingling warmth spread through my body, radiating outward from his touch. I lifted my arms, and he pulled the T-shirt over my head as we slid down onto the mattress.

6

"HOW DID YOU GET INVOLVED with dog mushing?" I asked Nick one day while we walked with our dogs through the woods.

"I answered an ad in a magazine," he said. "I was working in Arizona and I saw this job opening for a dog handler in Alaska. I thought it looked cool."

"No," I said, ducking under the branch he held up for me, "but how did you first get started—to get the experience to apply?"

Nick threw his head back and laughed. "Sweetie," he grinned at me, "that *is* how I got started. I applied."

Nick thought dog mushing should be an Olympic event. "It's just as athletic as any other sport," he'd contest to anyone who listened. "More so, in a lot of cases. Why should horse jumping be an event if dog mushing isn't?" This seemed, to me, a valid point.

Every time he described crouching over the back of a dog sled while flying down a black diamond ski slope into a hairpin turn, his eyes glowed as if his soul were on fire. "I got addicted to the adrenaline," he'd say, and I'd listen wide eyed and wondering how adrenaline addiction was possible.

"Why did you stop being a dog mushing tour guide?" I asked him one day. "You seem to really love it."

"I need to run my own team," he said. "It was time to move on."

I wasn't sure how I felt about dog mushing. Other than catching thirty seconds of coverage on TV or glancing at a random annual article about the Iditarod, I'd never paid much attention to the sport. According to Nick, there was a wealth of activity in touring, as well as sprint and mid-distance racing that took place across the globe. Now, compelled to think about it, I wondered how the sled dogs fared.

"Mushers love their dogs," Nick said, on the verge of bristling, when I brought up the subject. "We're all working for the same goal. I might be calling the shots, but I'm out there in the trenches right with the dogs." He described how mushers would run beside the sled when the dogs grew tired or to ease their load up a hill. "You wouldn't abuse your own team members," he told me.

I wasn't entirely convinced until he spoke of the bond he'd experienced with sled dog teams. We were sitting in the spacious foyer of his father's house in pea-green fabric chairs that squeaked when they rocked (because they probably were not meant to rock). We faced each other as we drank our coffee alongside the wall of windows opposite the front door. Nick's gaze shifted out the window to the expansive backyard. "There's nothing like it," he said. "You're part of a team in nature—you're part of the pack. Those dogs trust you with everything they've got. They trust you more than any person could." He looked at me. "I can't describe how it feels." He shook his head, stumped for words for the first time since we'd met.

Once, while we were lying in bed, I noticed a scar on Nick's stomach. "What's this?" I asked, trailing my index finger over the smooth, pale line.

"That's where I had my gall bladder out," he said. "I was seven years old. I think I was the youngest person on record to ever have that organ removed." It would, I thought then, have been the same year his parents had divorced. He laughed and curled his arm behind his head. "That was back when I still stuttered," he said. As usual, Nick was full of surprises.

Nothing stopped him from accomplishing his goals—not even his asthma, which I'd come to recognize as the worst case I'd ever known. He'd been diagnosed as a young child before inhalers came along and changed the way asthmatics could live. By the time he started kindergarten, Nick had already been rushed to the hospital, unable to breathe, on multiple occasions. He couldn't remember how many times the doctors had injected him with steroids to ease the inflammation that prevented oxygen from getting to his tiny, pre-K lungs.

I'd often hear him wheezing on our walks and sometimes as we lay in bed at night. I swore I felt my own lungs constricting as I listened to Nick's labored breathing—the steady sound of air trapped inside a taut balloon, pushing slowly through a microscopic pinhole to its freedom.

The idea that Nick would ever leave his house without an inhaler was incomprehensible to me. Yet he often did just that. We'd be walking through the woods or sitting in a restaurant when the familiar wheezing sound would commence. "Shit," he'd say, and I'd know that he'd forgotten his inhaler again. Nick's lack of precaution contributed to my belief that he simply had no fear. Up to that point, my basic understanding had been that life transpired inside of fear. As if fear were an elemental aspect of the atmosphere surrounding us—a bubble inside which we humans lived—and no decisions could be made nor actions undertaken without first consulting fear. If a person lived outside of fear, I wondered, could that person survive? In truth, Nick almost hadn't.

During one of the family reunions that his father hosted annually, Nick arrived without an inhaler. He was a teenager at the time—old enough to know better. Rather than drive him to the pharmacy, his father opted to teach him a lesson. In his struggle to breathe that day, Nick, as he described it to me, "blew a hole in" his lung. If his sister hadn't driven him to the ER, he may have died. He told me this without embellishment and little emotional expression. Just another average day on earth, his countenance seemed to imply. But in my mind, it was anything but ordinary. I never let on how much that story horrified me.

Holding those feelings inside may have prevented my coming to terms with them. I would always wonder what kind of a father would allow his son to suffer, let alone put his life in danger, just to teach him a lesson. For all the conflict I'd experienced in my family, I knew my parents would put their own lives on the line rather than take such a risk with mine.

For the first time, I considered the precarious foundation of Nick's life. He'd been seven years old when his parents split up and his mother moved him with his sister to Maryland, separated by an entire state from their father. Those circumstances upset his childhood stability. It happened quickly, from what Nick had shared, and I could only imagine the vast sense of unknown they'd all felt. At seven years old, such a deep unsettled feeling might settle in for good.

Where stability in my life meant having two feet on the ground, solidly fortified with deep, familial roots, stability for Nick may have comprised more of a balancing act. Perhaps his roots were not roots at all but a rubber ball on top of which he teetered, and balancing was easier as long as he kept the ball rolling. Perhaps Nick's stability was the moving ball beneath him.

Sometimes I thought I'd catch a glimpse of the childhood Nick—the little boy who still stuttered, lying in the hospital bed wide-eyed and terrified. I pictured seven-year-old Nick confused and hidden with his sister in the back seat of the car his mother was driving the night she stole out of town, having learned of her husband's infidelity with the next-door neighbor.

Ever since he'd asked for my phone number, I wondered what a person like Nick could see in a person like me. It occurred to me now that if I was attracted to his drive for adventure, maybe Nick was attracted to my roots.

7

ONE LAZY SUNDAY afternoon at my house, Nick cooked chili dogs. He diced up an onion as the chili simmered on the stove.

"Will you try some?" he asked, knowing I despised onions to the point of picking them out of my food. "Please?" He saw the hesitation on my face. "You have no idea how good this is."

"All right," I relented. My roommate had recently talked me into trying a few sautéed onions in our fried potatoes, and I hadn't instinctively purged. Maybe my tastes were changing. Nick held up his chili dog, and I leaned forward to take a bite. The pungent scent of body odor that I'd always associated with raw onions infiltrated my sinuses before assaulting my taste buds. I bit down and pulled a hunk of hot dog into my mouth. Nick watched my reaction, and I felt my face contorting progressively as I chewed. I willed myself to continue, determined to get the full effect in order to arrive at an educated decision. I shook my head back and forth unable to speak as I choked down the bite.

"I don't like it," I said, rushing to the sink for a glass of water. "Ugh. Ick. How can you like that?" Tears now clouded my vision. Nick laughed.

"I love that about you," he said.

"What?"

"That you'll try something. Even if you think you don't like it, you'll try it again."

"Well sometimes I change my mind," I said, wiping my eyes with a paper towel. The sharp flavor still permeated my mouth. I grabbed the bottle of beer he'd just opened and took a long swig. "Whew." I looked at him as I blinked away more tears and handed back his beer. "Don't ever make me do that again."

That night, we spread some blankets and pillows on the living room floor and watched *Holiday Inn*, one of Nick's favorite movies that I had never seen. The next morning, as we lay tangled up in my single bed, it hit me that we rarely went to the movie theater.

"Hey, we should go to a movie tonight." I said.

"I can't. I have to go to this dinner thing with my dad."

"Well, can't you get out of it?" I'd recently noticed that Nick rarely, if ever, said no to his father. This was a new and bewildering concept for me, as far as child-to-parent relationships went, and I was having trouble wrapping my head around it.

"No, I already told him I'd go." He rolled overtop of me to get out of bed.

"Where are you going now?"

"I have to work at Dad's hangar today," he said. Nick's father was paying him to do odd jobs while he was in town.

"I don't have to go to work until eleven. Why don't you stay for breakfast?"

"I don't have time," he said, pulling his shirt on and leaning down to give me a kiss. "My dad will already be there."

After Nick left, I stayed in bed, thinking about the extent to which his father seemed to be ruling his life. While I respected Nick's efforts to make money, I wondered if his father took advantage of their working relationship by controlling aspects of his personal life as well.

The longer I thought about it, the more I believed it, and I climbed out of bed to rattle off an email telling Nick exactly how I felt. What I received upon returning from work that evening was a digital diatribe of the most scathing personality critique I'd ever received. "You are spoiled by love," Nick's email began, continuing with a list of the many ways in which my family bent over backward to accommodate me and the many more ways in which I took advantage of those accommodations with little to no consideration for anyone but myself.

Granted, the dynamics in my family had shifted quite a bit over the years, and I supposed my parents did help me out a lot, maybe too much for a person my age. I couldn't afford a car on my salary, which barely covered rent and utilities, so my mother had permanently loaned me her car. And my dad remained practically on call, even when I didn't know I needed him.

When I first started working at the weather company, I was on third shift. I originally thought this would mesh well with my internal clock. If I worked overnight, I reasoned, my days would be free to hike with my dog, or to shop for groceries, or to do whatever I pleased. The detail I failed to recognize in this scenario was my status as a human being. We humans, it turns out, have to sleep sometimes. Typically, people sleep just before their respective work shifts. Mine started at 3:00 a.m. To get a full night's sleep before work meant I'd have to fall asleep at 7:00 p.m. This, in contrast to my original assumptions, directly conflicted with my natural tendency to stay up late. No matter what I tried, I could not get my internal clock to shift. I was lucky if I fell asleep at 10:00 p.m. Most often it was after 11:00, and I had to wake up for my work shift at 2:00 a.m. I'd come home exhausted, just before noon, when Katy would be wide awake and ready to start our day. We'd walk for a couple of blocks, but inevitably, I'd be too tired to hike or to shop, and whatever I pleased usually turned out to be napping until around 4:00 p.m., rendering it impossible to go back to sleep at 7:00.

I lost weight and, on top of my usual intestinal distress, developed acid reflux. My father noticed my weakened physique. He set me up with a hefty supply of Ensure to pump up my vitamin intake. This caused me to feel like a senior citizen and, at the same time, grateful that my dad still looked out for me.

I assumed such acts could make Nick think I was "spoiled by love." But I failed to understand how a person could get too much love. If Nick felt that way, why would he want to be with me at all? The reality slapped me across the face before kicking me in the gut, just to make sure there was no misunderstanding. My boyfriend thought I was a monster. This was the disaster I'd expected from the beginning. The fact that I could elicit such a visceral reaction with one email proved that I had no business trying to maintain a relationship. Apparently, I lacked a basic ability to communicate.

I printed Nick's response, filling four full pages, single-spaced, and I paced the halls of my house for days, reading and obsessing over his critical words. I did not call him. I did not email, and I did not expect to see or hear from him ever again. On the fourth day, he called me. I agreed to go to lunch, bracing myself for what I was certain would be our official breakup.

Nick picked me up in his Wrangler and, for the first time, Chief was not with him. We drove through town in relative silence and settled on a deli neither of us had tried before. Nick walked through the door behind me, and we chose a high-top table at the storefront window facing the street. He wore a faded baseball cap, the curve of its bill having been coaxed, over the years, into a tight, upside-down U. The whitewashed walls, counters, and tabletops made the restaurant brighter than the overcast day facing us on the other side of the window. I felt Nick watching me from across the table as the waiter walked over with menus. We placed our orders, then Nick launched the conversation that would determine our future as a couple.

"I know my dad is set in his ways," he said, "but he's done a lot for me. He's giving me a place to stay, and he's paying me to work for him. I've been away for a long time, and I have to spend some time with him while I'm here. I want to spend time with him."

"That makes sense," I said. "It just seemed like he's been making a lot of plans for you lately. I didn't mean to imply that you shouldn't spend time with your father."

"I know that isn't what you meant, but it's how it came across."

"Did you mean all those things you said about my family?"

"Look, you have a different relationship with your family than I have with mine. I just overreacted. I was angry, and I said some things I shouldn't have said." He looked down at the table.

"Do you want to break up?" I asked, looking into his eyes as he raised his head.

"I don't." Nick paused as the waiter brought our sandwiches to the table, giving me time to absorb his words. "I don't want to break up," he repeated. "I'm sorry for what I said. I really like your family, and you're lucky to have them."

"Well, I wouldn't go that far." I smiled. Nick's eyes softened.

This problem-solving method of calm and respectful conversation was new to me. When it came to emotional conflict, I had always believed pontificating lectures, screaming temper tantrums, and the unfailing silent treatment to be the only available tools. That day, as Nick and I ate our bagel sandwiches—his lox with cream cheese and mine turkey with provolone—he opened my eyes to the give-and-take system of mature communication. I took to it like an adrenaline junkie (now that I knew the condition was possible) might take to BASE jumping.

"I don't want to break up either," I said, then I paused. To apologize would be to admit that I'd made a mistake. I'd be exposing an imperfection. I'd be making myself vulnerable. I couldn't remember the last time I'd admitted to, or even accepted, being wrong about something.

"I'm sorry too," I said finally, gazing into Nick's deep brown eyes, and I knew I'd crossed a chasm into the next chapter of my life.

8

KATY SKITTERED AROUND at my heels as if she were in some sort of imminent danger, while Chief scoured the marble-tiled floor for scraps. Nick's father had invited me to dinner, and the dogs, as always, were confined to the kitchen.

"Here, Katy," Nick called, and she approached him slowly with her ears flattened against her lowered head. He'd been trying to get her to roll over for him, but she could not be coaxed. She submitted to his attention now, wagging her tail with her eyes glued to me as Nick stroked her back.

"I thought Anne was coming," I said, less for an answer than for something to say to Nick's father.

"She'll be here," he said, pulling open the massive door of his stainless steel oven to check on the ribs. The scent of char grilled steak wafted out.

"Those don't smell like barbecued ribs," I said to Nick.

"Dad does dry ribs," he said. "You'll love them."

Anne walked in as Nick and I were setting the table. "I got called in to work," she said and rolled her eyes.

"Surprise, surprise," I said. "They called me in for three shifts in a row last week!"

"That unlimited sick time policy sucks," Anne threw her purse on the counter.

"Here we go," Nick said.

"You try working for a company that barely pays you enough to survive and makes you sign a contract to keep you from going anywhere else!"

"All you two do is complain about that place. If it's that terrible, you should find a way to leave."

"There aren't that many other places to work in State College," I said. Lately I'd been exploring the local employment options. It was true that jobs, at least for a person with the limited skills in graphic art and design I'd learned by drawing weather maps, were hard to come by.

"There's the university," Nick said.

"I've been applying to that place for years," Anne said. "You have to know someone to get a job there."

"Dinner's ready," Nick's dad said, walking toward the table with a plate of steaming ribs. "Everyone sit down. I'll get the potatoes."

We gathered at the end of the twelve-foot table. The hard black top— either granite or marble, I presumed—matched the rock-solid floors. I hoisted the heavy metal chair closest to the island and appliances where Nicolas was preparing the rest of the meal. It scraped across the floor, and I squeezed against the table to sit down. Nicolas came to the table with a plate of baked potatoes, one for each, and a green salad that he'd tossed with oil and vinegar.

"Wow," I said, pulling the rib bone out of my mouth. "These are amazing. I've never tasted anything like it."

"I like them better than ribs with barbecue sauce," Nick said.

"So how are things going with your mom's website?" Anne asked.

Nick's mother was a full-time artist, and he was building a website to help her sell more work. He hoped the skills he acquired would translate into future income streams. His father's house served as a temporary home base, equipped with the office space and Internet connection he needed for his work. It also gave him the opportunity to spend time with his father in an unrestricted way he'd rarely experienced.

"Oh, you know," Nick said, cutting into his potato, "it's slower than I hoped. "But hey," he added with a chuckle, "we made one sale this week."

"I made a sale this week too," Nick's father cut in. He bit into a rib and tore off a sizable bite. "Found a machine for a guy," he said as he chewed, "seventy-five thousand dollar profit." He licked his thumb and tossed the rib bone to his plate.

"Ha!" Nick's head flew back and he clapped his hands. "That's great." He shook his head and sighed.

"Hey," his father said. "You could have had this business." Nick's father, from what I understood, had made his fortune buying and selling heavy equipment. "But you didn't want it."

"That's right," Nick said, "I had to save the planet instead."

I looked down at my plate to hide my smile.

After dinner, Nick and I washed the dishes then retired to his father's den where he'd set up his temporary office. I studied the maps he had laid out on the smaller desk facing the wall while Nick finished the work he was doing at his computer. He'd been researching western resorts to determine the potential for opening a dog sled touring company in any of the towns near those resorts.

"It's not looking good, sweetie," he said after a while, and I spun my chair around to face him. "The only state I can find with major resorts that isn't already saturated with touring companies is Utah."

"Oh," I said, sounding more negative than I'd intended.

"I know." He removed his glasses and slowly rubbed his eyes. "I'll keep looking."

That night we ventured out to a local bar for a couple of beers and a game of pool. The chill of the fading winter and energy of impending spring clashed in the evening air. Before the night was over, Nick dropped the bomb that I'd known for more than a year would be coming.

"We need to talk," he said in the way all dreaded conversations begin. I responded by looking down at the initials carved into the solid oak table at which we were sitting.

"I know," I said, trying to fortify the dam that was keeping all the water from gushing out of my eyes. I traced the letters with my fingers, wondering who had carved them and when.

"Hey," he said, reaching across the table to hold my hand. "I want you to come out west with me." I looked up as the dam gave way, and a rivulet of salt water traversed the contour of my cheek. The warmth of his soft brown eyes penetrated my heart. "I love you," he said, and a tidal wave gushed from my chest to my head. "And I want you to come." I searched his eyes and took a slow breath.

"You don't have to decide right now. I just want you to think about it. I can't stay here and do what I need to do with racing dogs. I have to move out west. I want to see where this relationship goes. But either way," he said, "I have to leave."

"When?" I said, my voice thick.

"It has to be over the summer," he said. "I need to get set up so I can start training dogs in the fall and be ready to give tours by winter."

"I thought you were going to race?"

"I am," he said. "But I need to make money, and giving tours is the way to do that. I'll start racing after I have the touring business up and running."

It all sounded reasonable. He needed to go. Where I fit in was not yet clear to me, and at the moment, I didn't have the capacity to wonder if it ever would be.

"I love you too," I said softly. "But..."

"Just promise me you'll think about it," he said, squeezing my hand as the droplet of salt water slipped from my cheek and disappeared into the crevices of the age-old initials in the table.

I promised.

9

I PROBABLY KNEW from the moment he asked that my answer to Nick would be yes. That I'd go with him out west or anywhere. Not because I was caught up in the excitement or romantic adventure of it. Just the opposite, by my own estimation. I was in this relationship for the long-term goal.

The idea of building a life with Nick and carving our future together filled me with hope. I didn't expect it to be easy, but we'd bear our struggles together. I would support him, and I knew he would do the same for me. In the process, we would grow our own roots.

Such was my rationale after weeks of deliberation. Had I been honest with myself, I'd have known right away; the reason I agreed to move out west with Nick was the simple fact that he wanted me to.

It would be another full year before we'd move, and in that time, Nick could not find a more opportune location than Utah in which to establish his dog sled touring business. The only thing I knew about Utah was that a lot of Mormons lived there—the same ones, for all I knew, who came knocking on your door at all hours of the day and night with their Bibles and their eighteen-year-old lifetimes of wisdom, trying to convince you that their religion is better than any you could have chosen on your own or with the help of anyone other than them. To top off that pearl of perception, I'd recently heard that the beer in Utah had a lower alcohol content than regular beer. Though such a rumor seemed unreasonable, somewhere I'd heard it, and it stuck to one of my more obsessive-compulsive synapses that I could not turn completely off. I fancied myself somewhat of a beer connoisseur, having been drinking the stuff for longer than I cared to publicly admit. By the age of twenty-eight, I'd worked my way up past the lagers and pale ales and into the oatmeal and chocolate stouts. I wasn't sure I could live in a place that boasted imitation beer.

Adding to that concern was a classic bout of stomach trauma that struck just over a month before we were scheduled to leave Pennsylvania.

I had learned to deal with my sporadic intestinal distress by resorting to a diet of Gatorade for as long as it took to reset my digestive system, but the treatment was far from foolproof.

Nick had received an invitation to an engagement party for his friend, Franco. The party would be at Franco's parents' home in Maryland, posing somewhat of a problem in my current physical state. I blamed the anxiety of the impending move for inciting the most prolonged and unmanageable intestinal episode of my life. My stomach ached all the time, and attempts to eat food ended in desperate dashes to the nearest toilet. Even the Gatorade I'd resorted to sipping as often as possible in attempt to keep myself hydrated failed to stay in my system long enough to perform its function. The last thing I wanted was for my cursed inability to control my anxiety to stop Nick from honoring one of his best friends. *Mind over matter*, I repeated like a mantra as the party date approached.

We made plans to stay overnight at Nick's mother's home, which was within driving distance of the party. I attempted to fast on the day of the trip, but upon our arrival, a mild cheese fondue with fresh baguette and a variety of seasonal fruits awaited. It was "just a light snack," Nick's mother insisted until I agreed to eat "at least a little something" before going to the party.

Nick and I were the first to arrive, and Franco's mother paused the margarita blender to greet us. As other relatives abandoned their respective food-preparation and party-arrangement stations to meet Nick's "new girlfriend," I felt a familiar pressure in my lower abdomen. *What a warm family*, I thought, ignoring my discomfort and semi-consciously contrasting this kindhearted family with my own. I smiled and joined the conversation to the best of my ability. The dull intestinal ache persisted, and I willed it away as someone handed me a freshly blended margarita.

Franco walked us through the sliding glass door to the patio, where his family had set up food tables and decorations for the party. The evening air hung heavy and still. A brightly colored piñata in the shape of a burro dangled from a branch in the lone backyard tree. Nick and I gave Franco the magnum of potato vodka we'd chosen as an engagement present, then I retreated to the sidelines as Nick jumped into the action to help Franco's family set up for the party.

Dusk descended as other guests arrived. I spotted Franco's fiancé, who was tall and blonde and supermodel beautiful, standing by the beverage table. I walked over to congratulate her on the engagement. As I slipped back into the evening shadows, I saw her pick up the behemoth bottle of potato vodka. "Ew," she scrunched her perfect nose. "I hate potato vodka," she said to the woman she'd just introduced to me as her sister. "You can't even taste it."

Franco's brother announced the start of the piñata contest, and everyone moved from the patio into the yard to gather around the tree. Several guests took turns at the piñata but none connected. Franco's brother handed Nick the long wooden stick, indicating his turn, then he tied the blindfold behind Nick's head. He spun Nick around three or four times, pointed him in the general direction of the piñata, and stepped away. Nick swung the stick with home-run force, but for all his enthusiasm, he could not find his target. After a few minutes, Franco's brother stepped in to help. Nick took one final swing, missed the pristine piñata entirely, and completed the valiant batting effort squarely on Franco's brother's right cheekbone—wood meeting flesh with a sickening thud. Franco's brother lunged to the side. Still wearing the gap-toothed grin he'd assumed to conquer the piñata, Nick turned toward the source of the thud and lifted his blindfold.

"Oh my God! Are you O.K.?" he said when he saw what had happened. "I'm so sorry." Several people stepped in to help Franco's brother, who promptly left the scene, I presumed, to find some ice or frozen peas or a porterhouse steak to put on that shiner, and the piñata contest disintegrated into the night.

Not long afterward, matter inevitably won over mind, and I rushed to find the nearest bathroom. By the time I finished, all my fears had been realized. The toilet would not stop running. I jiggled the handle three or four times (the only thing I knew how to do), but after ten minutes, I realized it was hopeless. The requisite second flush was out of the question. I considered my options. If I said nothing, the next person who used the bathroom might fix the toilet without incident. Maybe that person wouldn't realize I was the one who'd broken the nice Franco family commode. If events panned out differently, though, and people continued to use the toilet without knowing it was broken, things could get uglier.

The family had been so warm and inviting, and Nick had already broken one of their accommodating cheekbones. I could not, in good conscience, break the toilet too. I mustered all my courage to confess as I flung open the bathroom door, and there, in front of me, stood another brother—one with both cheekbones intact. With my head held high, in as casual a countenance as possible, I explained the toilet situation. It wouldn't stop running, I said. Plenty of toilets did that periodically, I told myself, as the eldest Franco brother smiled and nodded and assured me that the situation was under control. As he entered the bathroom, I skedaddled down the stairs, zeroed in on Nick, and told him I was very sick and needed to go back to his mother's house immediately, which was in no way askew from the truth. He drove me there then returned to the party. It was just shy of 10:00 p.m.

I spent the rest of the night and a good part of the morning in the bathroom. Nick returned from the party around 2:00 a.m. and fell asleep shortly after asking why I was still awake. I kept going, almost every half hour, until I heard his mother stirring downstairs.

"Sweetie," Nick said to me later that morning as I lay on the air mattress staring at the wall. "You have to go to the doctor." I didn't have the energy to explain my genetic anxiety issues.

"I know," I said.

"It's not normal to have all those stomachaches. I'm really worried about you."

"O.K." I said, and I closed my eyes trying hard to ignore the impending urge to go to the bathroom again.

My episodes had never been predictable. I'd suffered stomachaches as a child but didn't remember having problems in high school. I attributed later episodes to stress, assuming that my hormones had changed as I aged. My mother suffered from anxiety, though not in the same ways I did. Grammie's symptoms more closely mirrored my own, and she attributed those symptoms to anxiety. Therefore, I concluded, my problems were genetic.

When my anxiety struck, medication did not help. I'd tried Pepto, Imodium, Phillips, Tums—everything I could think of, and the Gatorade only served to replenish the electrolytes I lost through the near constant purging of each episode. I knew stress was the only rational cause, regardless of the fact that my problems did not always coincide with stressful events I could pinpoint. Further convoluting the issue was the fact that my problems always cleared up, as if by magic, with no indication as to how or why. I'd then push the conundrum of what had caused the problem in the first place from my mind until the next time an episode struck, which could be weeks, months, or years later.

I held off on calling the doctor for another week, hoping for a spontaneous ending to this most recent illness. But after losing weight for almost a month, I showed no signs of improvement. Coworkers invited me to their homes for weight-restoring dinners of cheese-stuffed ravioli and similarly carb-laden comfort foods.

"How are you feeling?" one such coworker asked, furrowing her brow as she stood to retrieve the bowl of hand-crafted ravioli from her kitchen counter.

"I feel fine," I replied, looking down at my dwindling pile of pasta "other than not being able to keep any food in my system." Another super-sized ravioli appeared on my plate.

"You need some good home cooking," she declared with a single firm nod of her head.

When I saw the doctor, she hesitated to label my condition, but she did prescribe medication she thought would help. It took another week for me to realize the medication did not help and, in fact, seemed to exacerbate the problem. Upon hearing this news, the doctor suggested I see a specialist, but the earliest appointment I could schedule was several months away. Factoring all the variables at hand, I deduced that one of two events would have transpired by that time: I would have wasted away to nothing or moved across the country with Nick. Either situation voided any reason to schedule the appointment, so I did not bother to call.

Instead, I concentrated on my upcoming move and tried not to think about the fact that my life felt out of control. I focused my attention on supporting Nick in his efforts to fulfill his dream. Ever since I'd seen the "New York City actors" perform *Man of La Mancha* at the summer-stock barn theater next to my hometown, I'd considered striving to achieve one's dream to be one of the most noble and worthy causes in the universe. The practical side of me relegated dreams to the category of luxury to be considered only after the basic necessities—like a mid- to high-salaried, full-time, 8:00 to 5:00, Monday through Friday job with health insurance (including dental and vision); a stable living environment sans platonic roommates; reliable and (fingers crossed) respectable transportation; and marriage, children, or pet options, per individual interest—had been secured. I was still working on the job part of the basic necessity equation, but my partner was ready to launch his dream. Chances were likely, I reasoned, that my own life would fall into place in the process of helping him.

10

AS THE DEPARTURE DATE with Nick grew near, I packed my belongings and scanned regional newspapers for graphic design positions in hopes of sending a resume or two out west ahead of me. I'd managed to send just one application before my computer, not even one year old, suffered a meltdown. Several days later, that computer—the tool intrinsic to my graphic design career—entered the IT emergency room to undergo extensive surgery. While awaiting the outcome, I continued to discard all expendables and pack only essentials for the trip out west and my new life in Utah. The job search, I was forced to put on indefinite hold.

"I have to tell you something," Nick said one day as I packed. He dug his hands into his pockets and shifted his weight where he stood.

"What?" I said, turning from the closet to face him.

"Sit down," he said, walking over to meet me on the bed. "It's my website business."

"I'll have to break up with you if you're dealing in porn," I joked.

"It isn't that." He looked at me. "Well, it's not what you think."

"What is going on?" I said.

He confessed that he'd found a way to make money that did, on some level, have to do with "adult entertainment." I tried to follow his explanation, but my limited knowledge of the Internet and possibly my state of shock blurred the details. His vague description brought to mind women posing topless, like those in a 1950s pinup calendar.

"It's not hard core," he assured me. "I would never do anything like that. And it isn't permanent. I just need to make some money to get started out west." The room spun around us as I looked into his steady eyes—the eyes with the lingering sadness. I trusted those eyes.

"I can't be with someone who exploits women," I said.

"It isn't like that. You know I wouldn't do that," and in truth, I didn't think he would. "I wanted to be honest with you," he said, "before we start a life together."

"I need some time."

"Look," he said finally, then sighed. "My mom always told me that the willow tree survives the hurricane by bending with the wind, but the oak tree fights against the wind and cracks in half."

"What the hell are you talking about?" I said.

"I really respect you for your values. But you never bend. It isn't realistic to think other people can live up to your standards all the time. Everyone is different. And sometimes, we just have to compromise."

I turned my face away from his and fixed my gaze on the floor. That's how I remained until dusk darkened the room, long after Nick had gone.

His words had left me deflated and ill, like I'd fallen from a tree house and knocked all the air out of my lungs. It took weeks to digest the information.

I now knew exactly what I'd been missing by not dating all those years during high school—the ability to compromise my values for the benefit of a relationship. Overcoming a challenge like this, I thought, would prove my commitment was strong enough to endure all that the future may hold. I'd always been told people deserve second chances, but I tended to be stingy in providing them. If I didn't learn now, I might never have a lasting relationship. Nick deserved this chance, I told myself, and I was no quitter. I would not abandon Nick, and I would not resign to another relationship failure by reneging on our long-term plans now.

The deflated and ill feelings faded in my resolve, and I adjusted to the new information by focusing on the fact that Nick's business would change as soon as he found a more admirable way to earn money via the Internet or through dog mushing. I respected him for earning his own money rather than relying on that of his father, and I could, to a certain extent, sympathize with his compromising a few values in order to do so. Life wasn't perfect, I'd grown to understand. This situation was only temporary. It was time for me to learn how to compromise.

In 1999, I drove my mother's 1988 charcoal gray Nissan Sentra wagon. Nick owned a navy blue, 1993 hard-top Jeep Wrangler, and he'd recently purchased an army trailer on which to build a dog carrier in anticipation of his future career. He would build the shell out of plywood before our trip and finish crafting the individual dog boxes inside after we settled in Utah. This way, we'd have more room to fit our combined possessions in the open box on top of the trailer, as well as in the hatchback of my handy Nissan wagon.

My parents scheduled an appointment for my car to undergo a full inspection before we left, and for once, I appreciated their precautionary tendencies. Dad met me at the mechanic's garage and drove me home after I dropped the Nissan off for its inspection. A few hours later, Mom called to break the news that the car had not passed. More importantly, the car would never pass an inspection again. The undercarriage had completely rusted out, rendering it unsafe to drive. It dawned on me then that my permanently borrowed car would not, as previously planned, carry me and my belongings across the country.

"Our family always did have bad luck," my mother said. She'd resorted to this phrase, or some variation thereof, more times than I could count over twenty-eight years of my life. Each time she said it, I felt as if she'd flopped a wet army blanket atop an already sizable pile on my back. The possibility of my crawling out from under the load diminished with each utterance of her assertion.

Dad devised a solution. He called his mother. Grandma owned a car she didn't use very often. It was a Pontiac and, as he'd suspected, she was willing to part with it for her granddaughter's cause.

Arrangements for the transfer would take time, so when Nick wasn't ready to leave on the date we'd planned, the ensuing events almost all worked out. The most significant glitch with this latest delay involved the time-sensitive issue of my expiring lease. On that order of business, Mom and Dad swooped to the rescue again, allowing me to move into their home with Katy and place my belongings in their storage unit. The potential for this brand of parental accommodation to inspire a "spoiled by love" accusation did not escape my attention, but I realized I'd take "spoiled by love" over temporarily homeless every time the two options presented themselves. I had hope that Nick, who was currently in Maryland celebrating a friend's hapkido graduation, might someday understand.

Not long after moving in with my parents, I received word that my computer was off of life-support, breathing on its own again, and I'd be able to pick it up in time for the trip. The reality of the impending cross-country move sank in with a surprising measure of relief. The puzzle pieces were in place. I had only to tiptoe through the next couple of weeks in my parents' house without detonating a land mine. Dad seemed content to avoid the subject of the move altogether, but Mom had never been one to suppress her opinions. She fired with precision, sometimes in rapid succession.

"What are you going to do in *Utah*? How are you going to make *money*? Why *Utah*? Well, *I* don't think it's a good idea at *all*," were some of the thoughts that launched from the depths of her diaphragm. It was true, Nick and I hadn't solicited alternative opinions with regard to the move. We were both twenty-eight years old, for crying out loud, and perfectly capable of making a mature and logical, life-altering decision on our own. After the first week, my mother adopted Dad's approach and stopped talking about the subject altogether, as if my plans were the result of a curse that would only come true if she uttered the dreaded word—*Uuutaaahh.*

Somewhere among the questions that flew like bullets and in the respite of their absence, my mother home-cooked all our meals like she did when I was young—a protein, a vegetable, and a starch—until I could get meals down and keep them there. Though I didn't regain any of the weight I'd lost, my stomachaches subsided. Still, my nerves had taken a toll.

My whole body had withered, and for the first time in my life I thought maybe I wasn't as tough as I'd always believed myself to be. Looking in the mirror, I realized I might actually be considered sickly. Even my bones seemed thinner. Just a few months earlier, I could barely wrap my thumb and forefinger the whole way around my wrist. Now I could do it with room to spare. So much for my hearty American, beer-swigging, ready-for-anything self-image. But if I wasn't the person I'd always considered myself to be, who was I? I wondered, not quite able to accept the sickly American, Gatorade-sipping, waiting-for-my-boyfriend-to-finish-his-partying-so-we-could-haul-our-lives-and-our-dogs-out-west-forever image.

Lucky for my self-esteem, Nick's timing had always been perfect. Just as all the negative aspects of my situation floated dangerously close to the surface of consciousness, he reappeared. The positive thoughts returned like floodwater forcing the nascent negativity into its proper place in the crannies of my subconscious. Nick was ready to go, and I felt free.

PART II
Mush

11

TWO THIRDS OF THE WAY through Indiana, Nick's voice crackled over the CB unit.

"We need to pull over at the next rest area," he said in a tone that snaked its way through the airwaves and settled in my chest like a boa constrictor.

Twenty minutes later, he sat beside me at the picnic table and gazed up at the thick clouds crawling across the sky. "The Jeep is breaking down," he said.

"But we're only in Indiana." I bit into my stale peanut butter sandwich and looked at Katy, whose food sat untouched beside her.

"I'm going to have to pull over when it starts giving me trouble from here on out. We'll have to stick together and keep the CBs on."

By the time we left the rest area, I was pretty sure Nick had told me everything there was to know about the fuel injection system in a '93 Jeep Wrangler, but I hadn't heard a word of it. For the last half hour, all external sound was blocked by the words buzzing around like house flies in my mind, *The Jeep is breaking down, but we're only in Indiana.*

Shortly after leaving the rest area, our CB units also went on the fritz. Transmission was so choppy and static filled that we turned them off altogether. We'd just crossed the border into Illinois when a toll area comprised of more lanes than I had ever witnessed in one location loomed before us. Corralled into a middle lane, I chose what seemed to be a reasonable course amidst a cluster of traffic emerging from the chaos. I looked around for the Jeep. Considering the vehicle's uniquely accessorized appearance, I presumed even a person like myself with limited powers of observation and some level of visual impairment would be hard-pressed not to notice the handmade wooden dog sled resting awkwardly atop the six-foot-high plywood cab built into a shimmering silver army trailer—all of which traveled behind, not to mention towered above, *The Little* Wrangler *That Could*. It was a sight to behold. It was a sight I hadn't beheld in at least twenty miles.

I picked up the pace, but after an hour with no Jeep sightings, I gave up the search and pulled into a rest area. I poured a bowl of water for Katy and was in the process of unfolding my AAA TripTik (courtesy of Dad), when Nick pulled up beside me and flashed his gap-toothed grin. He'd thought I was behind him and had been driving slowly so that I could catch up. Our opposing strategies negated all possibility of an en route sighting. I mustered a half-hearted smile at the miscommunication and subsequent serendipity of choosing the same rest area, trying, with little success, to accurately refold my map before getting back on the road.

Midway through Nebraska, I found myself pondering the probability that moving to Utah was a colossal mistake. We'd been driving in the same state for many more hours than it should have been possible to drive in a single state. Darkness had long since descended, and I was road weary. The confined solitude of my driver's seat provided plenty of time to dwell on the dismal state of affairs. With two dogs and everything we owned packed into our vehicles, we could not consider staying in a hotel. Also, we needed to conserve money. I'd been able to save around $2,000 for the move, but I knew nothing of Nick's financial status. It could not have been good, based on his most recent suggestion of driving down an isolated dirt road and spending the night in a cornfield. This idea conjured images of territorial farmers with shotguns, ready to protect their farmlands from wayward and potentially crop-damaging travelers. A corncob bed would not suffice. So on we drove through more Nebraska, looking desperately for anything resembling a campground. After sixteen hours on the road and several unsuccessful attempts at finding a campground with a vacancy, Nick posed another idea.

"How about sleeping at a rest area?" he said.

I considered the option in my frazzled state of mind and reasoned that, from an etymological standpoint, sleeping at a rest area sounded perfect. We continued driving in pursuit of this oasis, locating one mere moments, I was certain, before exhaustion rendered it unsafe to go on.

"Let's get our sleeping bags and put them on the tables under a pavilion," Nick said. The look on my face sent him back to the Jeep without another word, and I did my best to fall asleep in my seat, which could not recline for all that was packed in behind it.

Somewhere around 2:00 a.m., as I twisted and contorted in a vain effort to find a comfortable sleeping position with my dog wide awake in the passenger seat beside me and the entirety of my life's belongings crammed into the seat and trunk behind me, the gravity of the situation illuminated with sudden and fluorescent intensity. I had reached the kind of clarity that only happens in the mind of a sleep-deprived person during the wee hours of the morning. All the blanket-layered distortions of daily existence had dissolved, revealing the stark naked, indisputable truth. I was doing the wrong thing. Somewhere in the midst of this lucid cognition of my life-altering mistake, scrunched with my knees pressed into the steering wheel and my head lolled into the crevice between the seat back and the window, I fell asleep.

I woke up at 5:00 a.m., and then at 6:00. By 7:00, my joints ached so much from the contorted positions they'd been forced into all night that sleep was no longer an option. A haze clouded my early-morning mind, the clarity of a few hours earlier now fading into obscurity. I looked at Katy who had curled herself up in the passenger seat with her nose tucked under her leg. Her wide brown eyes stared at the air in front of her. I wondered if she knew where we were going—if her canine sixth sense had intuited the general direction of our path and surmised an approximate destination. This desert dog had not flourished in the desert the first time she was there, I remembered. Did she remember, too? I ran my hand along her back, feeling the protrusion of every vertebra, noting the surprising amount of fur that shed itself into my hand and floated through the air around us.

"You have to eat, K," I said softly, and she groaned in response, shifting her weight. "Your joints hurt, too. We've been cooped up in this car too long." I sighed and attempted to stretch as I glanced out the window at the Jeep and trailer parked across the lot with the RVs and eighteen-wheelers. I saw something move on top of the dog box behind the Jeep. I squinted, pressing my forehead against the window in an effort to see better, then Nick popped up from his previously prostrate position on top of the plywood cab. He'd slept on the dog box. *How in the world did he get up there?* I wondered before noticing he was grinning at me. He waved. I chuckled and prepared to emerge from confinement, ready to begin the new day with a candidly fresh perspective.

"Why didn't you sleep in the Jeep?" I asked as we sat at a picnic bench to feed and water the dogs.

"I wanted to stretch out," Nick said. "You should have come up. It was comfortable."

"Yeah, well, I didn't exactly know it was an option."

"You didn't seem too interested in options last night," he said, and the thoughts of sleeping in cornfields and on top of public picnic tables rushed back.

"I guess I wasn't," I said. I picked up Katy's untouched breakfast to prepare for another long day on the road.

With the Jeep in its compromised state, we drove less than forty-five miles per hour, stopping often to rest the Wrangler's weary engine. At no point in the journey was it clear that the Jeep would deliver us safely to our destination, but we did not consider alternatives. We lumbered along at this impeded rate, driving twenty minutes at a time with five- to ten-minute breaks along the way to improve our chances of eventual arrival.

While staying at my parents' house, I'd received a phone message regarding the single application I'd submitted prior to leaving Pennsylvania. A woman who worked for a real estate company in Park City said she'd reviewed my resume and asked me to contact her about the graphic design position when I arrived in the area. As far as I knew, that potential opportunity represented the closest thing Nick and I had to a plan. Because we didn't know when we might arrive, we had made no arrangements to meet anyone on a specified date. We'd brought the list of homes and apartments for rent that we'd printed before leaving Pennsylvania but had scheduled no appointments to look at them. We weren't even certain where we'd settle because Nick believed we'd have a better chance of finding a location and housing arrangement that accommodated his dog mushing-related requirements once we arrived. In the grand scheme of our new life, there was no reason to hurry. So we took our time along Route 80 West, stopping for one last night at a campground in Cheyenne, Wyoming, before continuing on into Utah.

We rolled into Park City in late afternoon as the sun drifted toward the horizon. I had never seen the likes of this former silver mining town built into a mountain—a city sitting on and surrounded by ski resorts. The homes looked like oversized dollhouses, petite and painted in decorative yet muted colors, like frosting on assorted sugar cookies. I smiled, suddenly feeling like I was on vacation. Good things were bound to happen in a place like this. We located the real estate agency at which I hoped to secure a job interview and, after a brief tour of the mountain paradise, descended into the Heber Valley in search of our final destination.

We found a tavern-style restaurant that looked nearly affordable about twenty miles south in Heber City. In standard fashion, Nick struck up a conversation with a man at an adjacent table. Though we had in our possession a list of rental units that were available as of the week before our trip, we would need a temporary place to stay. The man suggested a nearby state park that was likely to have some campsite vacancies. He gave us directions, and Nick and I clinked our pilsner glasses in toast to this good fortune. It was August 25, 1999. We'd made it to Utah and had found a temporary place to live. It's possible we'd have curbed our enthusiasm had we known that the Wasatch State Park Campground in Midway, Utah would serve as our primary residence through the better part of September.

12

DURING OUR FIRST WEEK at campsite #14, I learned rudimentary skills for pitching a tent, lighting a campfire, and cooking on a camp stove. Number 14 was a double site, which we chose for its spaciousness and close proximity to the full-shower- and flushing-toilet-equipped restrooms. This site offered a choice of two sand pits in which to pitch our tent, a fire pit for heat and cooking, a water spigot for washing up, and an extra long picnic table for which we had little use but that we considered a nice touch, anyway. It was no more isolated than the other campsites dotting the mountain around the one-way loop, but the scrub oak grew so thick and tall over the mountain that it blocked the view from one campsite to the next. Nick and I enjoyed our privacy those first few days. We'd find out that weekend just how popular the campgrounds were.

I'd camped in the past, though my girlfriends and I had clocked less tent time than anticipated on our trip out west in search of ski resort jobs. More nights than not, one of my friends had pleaded with a hotel desk clerk for a bargain basement rate on a room, and more often than not, this resulted in our sleeping indoors.

My longest stretch of camping had taken place during my exchange trip in college where, by some Australian magic, our science teacher (and would-be tour guide) had talked me into embarking on a seventeen-day bus tour through the Outback during the university's mid-semester holiday. Meals had been provided, as were associated campfires, and six years later, I'd forgotten anything tent-related I may have learned in that initial crash course. I did, however, recall feeling distinctly unnatural in the natural setting of Australia's Outback territory.

People change, I thought now, hoping my past camping experience might kick in to complete the outdoorsy persona that currently appealed to me. So far, I had to admit, things were starting off slowly. At least I'd learned the art of brewing a serviceable pot of coffee in Nick's battered aluminum percolator, which came in handy on those crisp Wasatch mornings when I awoke before he did.

Beyond the chill of those mornings, everything seemed crisper than it had in Pennsylvania. Since we'd arrived, the weather had been clear as a cardinal's whistle. It felt as if the atmosphere had been stripped clean out of the air. The sky boasted such a perfect shade of blue that it looked too good to be true—a color so sharp it could sting your eyes if you stared at it too long. This was raw, rugged air.

Utah's landscape also struck me as rugged. Most people called the mountains beautiful. To me, they were intimidating. Magnificent and humbling giants with razor sharp edges. I felt their unshakable presence at all times. Driving through the mountain passes made me feel small, like a microscopic insect that could be crushed at any moment without warning or regard. I found myself thinking that the odds toward injury or death were much higher in terrain like this than in the few other places I'd lived.

Nick had driven the Jeep into town for a tune-up the day after we arrived. This relegated my rusty but reliable Pontiac, recently named Betty Blue and still loaded to the roof with everything I owned, to the role of primary transportation for Nick, Katy, Chief, and me until who knew when. We'd rearranged my belongings, clearing enough back seat space to accommodate one large and one medium-sized dog, and had commenced exploring the scenic features and living options in the Heber City and Midway areas.

Referring to the list of rental units in our price range at $1,000 or less per month, we drove in search of addresses like 250 South 400 East, which did not seem complete to me. I expected the words east and south to appear as directional indicators for Park, or Maple, or any other street commonly named with a proper noun. It was months before someone informed us that all streets emanated in numeric intervals North, South, East, and West from the starting point of the Mormon Temple. Minus this critical clue, we wandered around the city in aimless hope of intersecting one or more of the streets on our list. Though this unscientific method required more time and mileage than a more systematic approach likely would have, it also came with the side benefit of familiarizing us with the nuances of our hometown-to-be.

We treated ourselves to local cuisine like dinner at The Claim Jumper and brunch at The Wagon Wheel, each time justifying the expense as a necessary product of research. We spent leisurely afternoons driving on back roads or strolling through the aisles of Smith's grocery store, just to soak in all the sights and smells of our fresh, new environment. Nick discovered the Alpine Loop Scenic Byway, a paved route through the alpine canyons of the Wasatch Range, which quickly became our favorite pastime. We'd wind our way through the switchback crack of a road nestled in the towering folds of deciduous-blanketed mountains to witness the shock of flaming colors that grew more vibrant with each trip.

For a while, this persistent state of exploration inspired me to focus on the promise of better opportunities. But reality has a way of illuminating the limits of possibility. After the third or fourth time Nick turned down a rental because it didn't come with a dog kennel or some other mushing-related problem, I realized our possibilities might not be endless.

Between excursions, I used the pay phone outside the park offices to schedule an interview with the real estate company in Park City. I had selected my most assertive while unassuming interview outfit—a pine green pants suit—and packed it neatly in a garment bag atop the boxes in my trunk, ensuring optimum accessibility, should this or any other company request an interview before Nick and I had fully settled. The rest of my wardrobe remained unattainable in the sealed end of the trailer nearest to the Jeep. At the accessible end of the dog box, Nick and I had organized a make-shift pantry stocked with the daily essentials—toiletries, food, and cooking utensils.

"You really have this camping thing down," I said to Nick one Sunday as he shimmied the pan in which our omelet sautéed over his camp stove and simultaneously swigged from his bottle of beer. It was another glorious Utah morning. The sun hadn't yet reached its peak, and temperatures were climbing into the 90s. "If it weren't for my bruised hips and shoulders, I might admit that camping can be comfortable." I rubbed my aching joints.

"Yeah, that sandpit is killer," he said. "We should go to Wal-Mart after brunch and buy an air mattress."

Any time we needed supplies we headed up the mountain to Park City, which suited me just fine because, so far, Park City topped the list of my favorite Utah locales. Sometimes we window shopped on Main Street or ventured into a gallery to look at jewelry or photography. Nick pointed out some sterling silver bracelets with Native American designs one day, and I made a mental note of the pieces he seemed most drawn to. I liked that Nick wore jewelry—another divergence from my previous notions of what men typically did.

Upon returning from Park City where, along with the air mattress, we'd picked up two folding camp chairs to secure our future comfort, we spread the mattress on the ground in front of the car then took turns blowing into it. Nick and I switched places only when we felt we might hyperventilate, carefully holding the plug for the other to step in before falling over and lying still to regain our senses.

"I'm gonna pass out," I said, inhaling deeply as I stared up at the piercing blue sky. It was the exact color of toilet bowl cleaner.

"You're gonna pass out?" Nick took a break from blowing, plugging the hole with his thumb. "I'm the one who has asthma," he reminded me before resuming.

"Oh yeah," I remembered. "Well my mom smoked when she was pregnant with me." Nick laughed, and a hissing sound emanated from the blowhole. "So my lungs are more than likely underdeveloped too," I assured him.

"This is fuckin' ludicrous," he said, half laughing, half blowing. I stood up to take my place at the head of the mattress and saw a neighboring camper walking toward us with something in his hand.

"Hello," I said. Nick turned around in greeting, his mouth still attached to the tube.

"I've been noticing you haven't gotten very far with that mattress," the man chuckled. After thirty minutes of blowing, there was barely a discernable rise in the inflation level. "I have this air pump if you want to borrow it," he said, extending the hand that held the pump. "It hooks right up to your car."

Nick's jaw dropped, and the tube fell out of his mouth. "Sure!" he said. "That would be great."

"My wife just drove the car into town. Would you mind if I brought my mattress over here to blow up?" the man asked.

"Of course not," I said.

"No problem at all." Nick took the air pump and hooked it up to my car as the man left to retrieve his mattress.

The remainder of the process took about eight minutes, not to mention significantly fewer brain cells. And the quality of our sleeping setup substantially improved after that. Not only did the air mattress relieve our aches and pains, but it also kept us warmer by serving as a barrier against the cold surface of the earth. Even a seasoned outdoorsman like Nick was beginning to suffer the chill of September nights in the high desert mountains. I snuggled against him to stay warm and, I hoped, safe against the gaping wilderness that surrounded us.

We were still living at the campgrounds when the time came for my interview at the real estate company in Park City. I met with a woman named Sue who greeted me with a firm handshake and a friendly smile. She wore khakis, a denim button-down, and a suede vest. She spoke directly and exuded an overall salt-of-the-earth countenance that made you trust her like an immediate friend. With deep brown eyes and the reddish tan skin of the desert, Sue looked like the pioneer version of Diane Lane. I learned she was the marketing director for this company which, she somehow explained in a way that diluted the intimidation potential, was the largest real estate company in Park City, Utah. We talked about my work experience. I showed her my portfolio. We conversed with comfortable ease and, for a moment, I had hope.

"How can I get ahold of you to set up a second interview?" Sue asked in conclusion, and I paused.

"I'm sort of in transition right now," I said, my mind spinning to come up with a reasonable solution in my homeless and phoneless state of existence. "Would there be any way that I could call you?"

"Sure," Sue said. "Let me get you a card."

I was still grinning in disbelief halfway down the mountain toward the campground when reality jolted my memory. Clothes. I hadn't anticipated a second interview. Everything I owned other than jeans and a fleece was buried six feet deep behind everything Nick owned in the extreme back end of a homemade plywood dog box. I wouldn't know which to extract for another interview outfit even if I *could* reach my suitcases.

"What am I going to do?" I said after returning to the campsite and explaining the situation to Nick. My breath quickened as the panic rose to my chest, pressing against my lungs.

"Sweetie, it's O.K.," Nick put his hands on my shoulders to stave my impending hysteria.

"How can it be O.K.?" I screeched. "I can't afford to buy another interview outfit!"

"We'll find something in the truck. I'll unpack some stuff and pull out your suitcases."

"My clothes are so crammed in back there. They'll be all wrinkled and ruined..."

"They won't be ruined. Tara, we'll figure something out. Let's just try." He looked at me with his steady gaze. "What else can we do?" he said. I stopped to consider the answer, and my panic leaked out in a long, slow breath.

The next day, Nick helped me empty the entire dog box to find my suitcases beneath the layered heaps of our belongings. I located another interview outfit and pulled out a few more comfort items while I had the chance—a hair dryer and an iron to smooth out my newly excavated suit. We had finished repacking the dog box and were perfecting our pseudo pantry when a park ranger appeared and told us we had to move. The campsite in which we currently resided was rented for the weekend. If we wanted to remain at the campground, we'd have to find a different site.

Considering our limited options within a 2,000-mile radius, we chose campsite #26, one of the few still available for the weekend. Nick made arrangements for the park ranger to move the trailer and dog box for us, since the Jeep was still out of commission. We broke down the tent, carried it across the campground, and pitched it back up in yet another sand pit. Remembering our ordeal with the air mattress, we agreed to take measures—extreme if necessary—to avert any situation that would require re-inflation. We each hoisted an end and carried the fully inflated queen-sized mattress around the looping road to our new campsite. As we rounded the bend with our exposed mattress in hand, a light drizzle began to fall. We would move in similar fashion three times during our stay at the Wasatch State Park. It would rain every time.

As Labor Day weekend approached, the Wasatch State Park rangers made it clear that Nick and I would have to vacate the premises. The campgrounds, they informed us, were fully reserved from Saturday through Monday to accommodate attendees of an annual festival in Heber City that drew 100,000 people from miles around.

"Heber City couldn't hold 100,000 people if they were stacked on top of each other," Nick said to me privately. His research on the city showed a population of less than 7,500. But our skepticism failed to negate the fact that we did not hold one of the coveted weekend reservations. We considered splurging for a hotel but agreed to hold off on that decision until the weekend arrived. The campground was bound to have at least one cancellation, Nick felt certain.

Earlier in the week, one of the park's office workers had stopped him at the gate. She had mentioned to a friend that a man with a dog sled was staying at the campground, and the friend turned out to be a woman Nick had contacted before we left Pennsylvania. Her name was Rose, and her brother had been a well-known sprint racer in the dog-mushing world. When Nick originally spoke with Rose, she'd had no rental space available. We now learned, through the Wasatch State Park office grapevine, that Rose's nephew and his girlfriend planned to move out of the mobile home they currently rented from her. Nick contacted Rose again, and she invited us to look at the rental, which was located next to her house in Midway, she told us, on Stringtown Road. Finally, a street with a name I could grasp.

The sun beamed over the farmlands lining Stringtown Road as we approached our potential new home. An enormous metal Quonset hut reflected the sunlight off to our right, and what looked like a large elm tree rose from the front yard on our left. The mobile home sat behind the tree, anchored to the earth by a plywood porch topped with artificial grass carpeting. Brown shutters and porch beams accented worn yellow siding, and the entire display, with its crooked components, rested in resolute conviction, like an octogenarian perched on his porch to watch the days pass until no more days come to pass. This mobile home, it was clear, had nothing left to answer for.

Nick stared straight ahead as Rose led us inside. Her nephew currently lived in the home with his girlfriend. He was a stone mason, Rose told us. He had constructed a solid concrete slab on which to position the woodburning stove, which he'd cornered in with one full wall and another half wall of river rock. The handiwork was so perfect that Nick and I took it for some kind of 1970s plastic facing until we noticed the floor. While the rest of the mobile home appeared to be made of materials no stronger than particleboard, the corner with the stove was visibly sinking under the weight of the concrete slab and solid rock wall. We touched the sea-shell-colored stones. They were perfectly smooth and absolutely real.

Walking through the rest of the rooms, we noticed the current residents' orderly presentation of densely accumulated belongings. Under different circumstances, this observation might have inspired us to question the couple's relocation timeframe. (As it turned out, they did not have one.) But the days were growing shorter and the nights notably colder. The encroaching winter reduced our faculty for logic on this topic.

Rose sweetened the deal by telling Nick that, for an extra forty dollars a month, he could use the barnyard across the street as his dog kennel. When she said she'd throw in three sled dogs left over from her brother's team, they sealed the deal with a handshake. We could move in as soon as the current residents moved out, Rose told us, though she had no idea when that would be. She did, however, have intimate knowledge of the Labor Day festival coming to town that weekend. Realizing Nick and I might not have a place to stay, she offered to let us pitch our tent in her yard or set up residence in the Quonset hut across the street from her house. We thanked her for her generosity and hoped the situation would not warrant such primitive extremes.

Nick picked up his Jeep from the repair shop before our Friday campsite eviction, as there had been no cancelations at the campgrounds. While the extra space made traveling more comfortable, it did not aid in the attainment of our goal to find adequate weekend shelter. We drove for hours in what was, by my estimation, a genuine monsoon, looking for a hotel, motel, inn, or bed and breakfast vacancy before resorting to Rose's offer.

We swept at the layers of silt-like dirt on the Quonset hut floor, shifting the prevailing odor from that of wet cow to stale manure in the process. After pitching our tent on the concrete floor, we found the canvas camp chairs we'd bought on inspiration at Wal-Mart and set them up at the mouth of the Quonset hut facing the open fields across Stringtown Road.

The sky darkened with cumulonimbus clouds that billowed like the mushroom pillows of nuclear explosions discharging straight from heaven. Lightning threaded through the clouds and thrust into the distant mountains in electric daggers of blue and gold, and the thunder rumbled from above as if it expected the mountains to answer back. When they did not, it grew louder.

In the same instant I realized what a privilege it was to be witnessing such a raw and uninhibited display of nature, I hoped the storm didn't move any closer to our scantily sheltered location. It was magnificent and humbling, and when it was over I saw colors of the universe I hadn't known existed. The clouds parted just above the mountain range before us, and as the sun's rays fought their way through the dense haze, filaments of gold glittered and hung suspended in the air. The sun was about to lose its battle for the sky as dusk crept over the Wasatch range behind us, trapping the golden refractions of light in the center of this now silent war between night and day. My eyes glazed over, and I thought I saw a giant bird land in the field across the street. The grass was so high that I wasn't sure I'd seen anything at all until more giant birds floated in from the sky. Before I knew it, there were fifty of them. I had no idea what they were.

"Sandhill cranes," Nick said before I had a chance to ask. "I saw them here yesterday."

"What are they doing here?" I asked.

"Migrating." He looked at me. "Dummy," he said with a dopey voice and his gap-toothed grin. I continued to stare at the birds, who were now making quite a ruckus. A cacophony of flugelhorns, I thought. My dad used to play the trumpet. I hadn't thought much about home since we'd left. I wondered what my parents were doing at that moment. I wondered if they were wondering about me.

13

NICK AND I AWOKE to sparkling skies and agreed to spend our morning with the new sled dog team. Shane, Midnight, and Shy lived in a covered area of the barnyard just behind the Quonset hut. These jet-black, short-coated dogs comprised of greyhound, Irish setter, and some breed of hound for speed and stamina, stayed behind when the men of the family—including Rose's dog mushing brother—rounded up the cattle and moved south where the grazing land was apparently more affordable.

We had no idea how long these leftover sled dogs had been chained in the barn before we arrived. Rose's brother had bred the dogs himself and was apparently known for his sleek black pack. Shy was the smallest of the three and, judging by her name, came by her timid disposition naturally. Shane and Midnight were brothers, around fifty pounds each and as loveable as teddy bears, though Shane took the prize for most affectionate.

I could get attached to these dogs, I thought as I stood on the receiving end of one of Shane's signature bear hugs. He stood on his hind legs with his two front legs wrapped around my torso, and I hugged him back and scratched behind his ears, content with how different my life was now than it had ever been before.

Here I was in the middle of the high desert, 2,000 miles away from my mother's proud house and about to start living with a bunch of dirty, smelly animals. I scratched the length of Shane's back, feeling the grime from his coat build up under my fingernails as he leaned against me and groaned with canine pleasure. *Life is good*, I interpreted that groan to mean. "Shane," I said, inhaling the musty barnyard air, "I couldn't agree more."

Around lunchtime Nick and I hopped in the Jeep to go check out the festival that had stirred the whole town into a frenzy. Swiss Days, people were calling the outdoor event, and, though local reactions implied something more grand than I could imagine, I looked forward to doing something as familiar as an arts and music festival. Every July since I could remember, State College had hosted the Central Pennsylvania Festival of the Arts—a four-day street fair that supplied my annual infusion of culture. I felt, somehow, at peace among the eclecticism of such music and art festivals.

Driving through Heber City toward Swiss Days put me in mind of what it might be like to drive in Midtown Manhattan on New Year's Eve. The road had been reduced to one lane as a result of the parked car overload along each side. Herds of people had turned the driving lane into their sidewalk, slowing traffic to an unreasonable pace. Homeowners along the route held up signs listing the cost to use their yards as parking lots, and we were still a mile away from the festival. When I suggested we pull into someone's yard, Nick said he'd rather spend the afternoon in the manure-infested Quonset hut than drop twenty dollars to be blocked into a backyard a mile away from our destination. We snaked our way to the edge of the festival, where Nick squeezed into a slot between a dumpster and a pine tree behind a corner booth.

From what I could tell, the festival grounds didn't cover much more than a city block, despite its 100,000-person draw. The crowds surpassed my comfort zone, but I overcame my uneasiness in the quest to experience some authentic Swiss culture. I noticed an abundance of the usual American craft suspects—wooden ducks and dried flower arrangements along with pastoral pink and country blue wall hangings featuring rhymes or traditional words of wisdom. I wasn't sure if such decorations represented Swiss culture or not, but I'd seen strikingly similar effects at many Pennsylvania Dutch-inspired festivals back home. I did see clogging and yodeling on the entertainment schedule for later that afternoon, and I wondered if those represented some of the Swiss traditions I'd expected Swiss Days to deliver. My stomach growled, reminding me that we hadn't eaten lunch, and I suggested to Nick that we look for something Swiss to eat before taking one more step toward the Santa doll stand.

The first food we encountered was a ham and Swiss cheese sandwich vendor. Next to that, we watched a girl with blond braids and a red and white striped cap distribute brightly colored scoops of ice in familiar cone-shaped cups through the window of a stand labeled "Swiss Ice." After exploring similar options, we settled on lunch at the "Swiss Navajo Taco" joint. I had never heard of this potential treat, but it wasn't long before Nick informed me that Navajo tacos represented fairly standard western fare. Apparently the "Swiss" version was no different than any other Navajo taco available this side of the United States.

We wouldn't stick around for the yodeling or the clogging, having consumed our fill of "Swiss" culture with the taco experience. The crowd was thickening, and in the hot sun, people seemed a bit irritable. By the time we left, so were we.

Nick had wanted to build a few simple pieces of furniture since we'd thrown away all belongings that would not fit in our cars and trailer prior to the trip. We both agreed that making furniture represented a more productive way to spend our Saturday afternoon than watching an alleged Swiss person clog. We drove to Lowe's in Park City where Nick found everything we would need to craft two identical bookshelves.

Back at the Quonset hut, he cut each board to size using the table saw he'd brought from Pennsylvania, and I did my best to sand the boards down before he assembled the pieces. The day was hot, and the work slow going and frustrating. After a couple of hours, we took a beer break and sat in our camp chairs at the mouth of the Quonset hut. The depressing fact was that the rumor had been true. Utah beer did, indeed, have a lower alcohol content than its otherwise identical relatives in practically any other state. I would make it my mission in Utah to find out why, I thought, as I sipped my two-percent alcohol content Beck's. It was still surprisingly refreshing.

We were hot and tired and lazy, and we gazed across the road at two people working in the garden across from us. They noticed us staring. The woman held what appeared to be a world record-sized zucchini in her hand and waved it over her head in our direction. The man was a giant. I wondered if he had descended from Vikings, then I realized that he must be the stonemason. The people across the road were the current residents of our future mobile home. We continued to stare.

"Do you want some zucchini?" The woman bellowed from fifty feet away. Shocked out of our reverie, we looked at each other, then back at her.

"Uh," I stammered.

"Sure," Nick yelled, and we leapt from our camp chairs and started across the road. Normally we would have expected the initiator of the conversation to walk over to us, but on this occasion, the woman waving the zucchini had only one leg.

"You want some zucchini?" she said again, at roughly the same decibel after we'd reached the yard.

"Sure, we love zucchini," I said.

"That's quite a zucchini," Nick laughed. It was at least a foot and a half long and six inches in diameter. "I'm Nick," he said.

"And I'm Tara."

"It's nice to meet you," the man said.

"We've got lots of 'em," said the woman. "You're welcome to have some." She leaned on her wooden cane to step toward us and hand over the super-sized vegetable.

"Thank you. That's really nice of you," I said.

"So how long are you staying in the Quonset hut?" the man asked.

"Just until Monday afternoon when the campground clears back out," Nick said.

"Well, we're fixing up the house there." The man pointed to the split-level home across the garden from the trailer. "That's where we'll be moving once it's ready. You're welcome to use the bathroom in there this weekend if you need to."

Nick thanked the couple for their generous offer while visions of powder room privacy danced unrestrained in my head. It had been weeks since I'd used anything other than a public restroom. While Nick talked, I scanned the enormous garden that this couple had been harvesting. There were huge pumpkins and squash, corn, and a colossal sunflower patch, in addition to the prolific zucchini. As the conversation drifted into farewells, that one beautiful thought returned to the forefront of my mind. *A real bathroom to use for a whole weekend.* This luxury seemed too good to be true.

Later that evening, I would fulfill the "too good to be true" prophecy by clogging our new neighbors' toilet and flooding the entire room. As I groped to turn off the water valve, my mother's assertion of our chronic bad luck consumed my thoughts. I found a roll of paper towels in the bathroom closet and sopped up most of the mess. *How many toilets across America am I destined to break?* I asked myself, wondering if our new neighbors—our only potential friends in the entire state of Utah—would ever speak to us again. *What the heck were their names?* I wondered before returning to the Quonset hut with my humiliating news.

I told Nick we'd better treasure our one zucchini because there would probably be no more where that came from. "And by the way," I continued, in hopes of steering his mind away from the subject, "I can't think of their names. Do you remember?" Nick looked stumped.

"I have no idea."

"I don't think they told us," I said.

"No, they definitely didn't."

"We should call them Gardenias," I said, "because of their gigantic garden."

"Hah!" Nick clapped his hands and flung his head back in laughter. "I wonder what they're gonna call us!"

Memories of the water-logged bathroom flooded my head, and I cringed in an effort to wring them back out.

When Monday rolled around, I heard the words "I can't wait to get back to the campground" fly out of my mouth before I consciously recognized what I was saying. I never thought I'd so much as think it, let alone say the words out loud, but we'd been living in the Quonset hut without a working bathroom for two days. In addition to dwelling among the grime and stench of a barn, we'd spent a lot of time with the barnyard dogs who, for all we knew, had never had a bath in their two years on earth. Our skin crawled, and we smelled like dirt.

Nick was up with the sandhill cranes around daybreak that morning. When he came in to wake me, sometime after 8:00, he'd already told the Gardenias about the unfortunate event in their soon-to-be-new bathroom.

"What did they say?" I asked, on the edge of my air mattress.

"They said that bathroom didn't work very well to begin with. They were planning on fixing it when they moved in."

"What?"

"They were cool." This was outside my realm of comprehension.

"They weren't mad?"

"Not at all."

I assumed he was protecting my feelings, but the sugar-coated version was O.K. by me, especially if it saved me from the humiliation of breaking the news myself. I should have remembered that taking the easy way out had never meshed with my nature. This fact hit me later that day when I spotted our future neighbors working in their yard, and my guilt compelled me to walk over and apologize in person.

"It's O.K.," they both said.

"The toilet didn't work all that well anyway," the man continued. "We're redoing the whole bathroom when we move in." Nick had been right. These people were amazingly laid back.

"Well, thanks," I said. "I'm sorry anyway."

"Don't worry about it," they said in unison, not even cracking a smile at the nature of the damage I'd done. "It's no problem."

14

WE RETURNED TO OUR CAMPSITE of choice, luxurious #14, shortly after 4:00 p.m., and I indulged in a world-record-length camp shower. Freshly scrubbed and feeling once again human, Nick and I contemplated our options for cooking the mammoth zucchini the Gardenias had bestowed upon us that weekend.

"We could make spaghetti with zucchini sauce," he suggested, and, though I'd never heard of zucchini-laden pasta sauce, my curiosity about cooking spaghetti over a campfire spurred me to agree to the challenge.

By the time we returned from the grocery store with ingredients, the sun was sinking in the sky. We wrapped a chunk of zucchini in aluminum foil and threw it on the hot logs at the edge of the fire. As that steamed, we placed a pot of water in the flames to boil and dumped a jar of Ragú into our frying pan. We added the zucchini to the sauce once it began to soften, then heated it all together over the flames.

Nick's campfire cooking expanded my culinary horizons. He never let obstacles, like the Jeep breaking down during our trip, get in his way. I knew he'd keep us safe in the wilderness and eventually succeed in forging a domestic home for us. I don't think he considered other options, such as those that flitted sporadically in and out of my own mind: *what if I don't get a job?* or *what if we don't find a place to live?* or *what if we run out of money?* The list grew daily. Believing in Nick seemed a better option than succumbing to my speculations on the various ways we could fail. So I left the planning and decision-making to him. This pioneer-style life was Nick's area of expertise, not mine, I thought as I watched him prepare our meal.

"I'll make chocolate pudding for dessert if you want," I said, and a grin crawled across Nick's face.

"Chocolate pudding," he said in a boyish voice. Nick always wanted chocolate.

We stuffed ourselves so full of food that after the meal, neither of us wanted to move. As dusk dissolved into dark, I leaned back in my camp chair with Katy's leash resting loosely in my lap, and I stared into the fading flames of the campfire. My gaze deepened, and I lapsed into the familiar food-induced stupor of overindulgence. The scent of smoldering logs combined with a touch of Grandma's home cooking in the faint aroma of spaghetti sauce still lingering in the crisp, night air. My eyelids slid halfway shut.

"Chief!" Nick yelled, and I jerked upright as a mad scuffle arose in the dark off to my left. Before I knew what was happening, I was on my feet screaming and lurching toward my loose dog. It happened so fast—the dogs running, the chase, the barking and yelling, and then the scent. The burst of nostril-burning rancor that stood time still for a flash, then exploded into a slow-moving cloud over our camp world and beyond. Inside the noxious cloud, time slammed on the brakes, and in my dreamlike state, I groped for the flailing leash, grasping it milliseconds before Katy crossed paths with the direct stream of olfactory venom. Chief, leashless and first on his feet, was not so fortunate.

I pulled Katy under the camp spigot before noticing Chief's reaction. He pawed at his face, shaking his head while sneezing and snorting like he'd inhaled a swarm of killer bees. When that course of action failed, he pushed his face into the ground, rubbing each side against the gravel before Nick took him by the collar and guided him to the main park showers for a full-on soaking.

We'd heard the Wasatch State Park skunks scavenging in the fire pit the week before, but they usually emerged well after dark when the only havoc they could wreak was that of thwarting my late-night trips to the restroom. They must have grown accustomed to the extra garbage left by campers that Labor Day weekend. Tonight, the skunks stamped their padded feet, in presumable irritation at our ruining their dinner, before meandering out of the campsite and back under the cover of surrounding shrubbery. Chief looked at me with glassy eyes, as if to ask what just happened, and my heart went out to him before the true source of his confusion occurred to me. The skunks were gone, and all Chief likely wanted to know was, *Which way did they go?*

The next day I realized we all stank. This was problematic in relation to the second interview Sue had asked me to schedule that week with the president of the company. I held off on calling for a few days, thinking the refreshing Utah air might whisk away the majority of the negative odor. Perhaps if any scent lingered, it would be mistaken for earthy rather than skunky, which I hoped would be acceptable given our rustic, western location.

When I called to schedule the interview, Sue wasn't available. I waited several more days before trying again, securing as much extra time as possible before the in-person meeting. We finally scheduled the interview for the following week. The president, Sue told me over the phone, was also the owner of the company. Standing at the payphone outside the Wasatch State Park ranger's office, I glanced up the mountain toward the campsite which served as my current home, and I realized that nothing short of a miracle would land me that job.

I spent a lot of time hoping for a miracle that week. When the interview day came, I spread a bath towel over the hood of my trusty blue Pontiac upon which I ironed my trusty tan pants suit in a tenacious effort to help my not-so-trusty miracle grow to fruition. I started up the mountain toward Park City with my hair still wet from the shower, hoping the saturation would accentuate the smell of my pomegranate shampoo as opposed to any other odor that might be lingering in the recesses of my follicles.

The owner of the company carried the air of a successful one-man show. His swept-back hair looked like freshly fallen snow, framing a face that years of experience had molded into the picture of self-possession. Ice-blue eyes studied my every response. Signs of rapport in those eyes were fleeting, and for the most part, this company owner and president appeared less than impressed. To wrap up the interview, he asked about my origins. This triggered a conversation about my trip out west to support my boyfriend who, I told him, planned to be a dog musher. His eyes softened as he reminisced about coming to Utah with his wife many years earlier. He'd found his success in Utah, he told me. *A swing and a hit!* I thought. He and his wife had since divorced, he said. *Stee-rike.*

We shook hands, and I smiled as pleasantly and maybe as desperately as possible. I would take pity at that point. Sue told me to give her a call the following week, as my extended state of "transition" would prevent her from reaching me with a final decision. A butterfly fluttered through my stomach, and I raised my hand to settle it. As long as I could avoid the failure pit, I knew I'd be safe from the anxiety-induced trauma I'd suffered before leaving Pennsylvania.

"How'd it go?" Nick asked when I returned to the campsite.

"O.K.," I said. "Not so great."

"I'm flying back to Maryland for Franco's wedding next weekend," he reminded me.

"I'm getting a motel room," I said, staring into the woods.

"I think you should." He handed me a beer. I took the bottle and sank, still clad in full second-interview regalia, into my ten-dollar Wal-Mart camp chair.

One more week of camping. Two more campsite changes. Seventeen hundred calls to Rose to find out when we could move in to the non-mobile mobile home. Finally, an answer. The Gardenias, who by that time we'd learned went by the names Dan and Kelli, would be moving out the weekend Nick was flying back to Maryland. We could move in the Monday he returned. The end was finally in sight, I thought, and so was the beginning.

We officially moved out of the Wasatch State Park, and Rose was kind enough to let us stash our belongings in the Quonset hut while Nick traveled. I found a motel for less than $50.00 a night that permitted Katy, as a medium-sized dog, to stay in the room. Large-breed Chief would have to stay in the barnyard with Shane, Midnight, and Shy. I'd visit to feed and water them every day and to let Chief run free and stretch his legs, which were not accustomed to the chained restraint of a six-foot circumference.

In the motel room, I flipped on the television then retired to the bathroom for a lengthy shower. Katy was fast asleep on the bed when I emerged. I flopped beside her and cycled through TV stations, landing on coverage of the US Open. My mother had taught me how to play tennis in college, and we often watched the Grand Slam tournaments together. I placed the remote beside me and settled in.

At 4:00 p.m. I peeled myself off the bed to use the pay phone on the sidewalk at the edge of the parking lot. First, I called Sue at the real estate company to inquire about the job. They hadn't made a decision yet, she told me, and I released the breath I hadn't known I'd been holding. It would probably be best not to call again until Nick and I were settled, I thought, still gripping the receiver in its cradle. I picked it back up and dialed my parents. "Hold on," my mother said. "Your dad wants to pick up the other phone."

I told them Nick had flown to Maryland for his friend's wedding, so I was now staying in a motel room.

"Are you calling from the room?" Dad asked. "Give us the number, so we can call you if we need to."

"There's no phone in the room, Dad. I'm at a pay phone."

"Did you hear about the job yet?" Mom asked. The question shot through my chest like a bullet.

"They haven't made a decision."

"Well, when will you know?"

"I have no idea. How are things at home?" I changed the subject.

"Good, good, they're fine," Dad said.

"Are you watching tennis?" Mom asked.

"Every second. I haven't seen TV in so long that my eyes are glued to it. It's like a luxury just to have a TV and a bed." Even better, I neglected to mention, was the proximity of the bathroom. Gone were my flash-lit nights of dodging past skunks and unknown critters and trekking fifty yards to a cold, dark, isolated building to relieve my bladder before going to sleep.

"When do you move into your new apartment?" Mom asked.

"Monday. I'll let you know when we're settled." The conversation dwindled.

"Call again tomorrow with an update," Dad said.

"Dad, I can't call every day from a pay phone." The edge in my voice sounded sharper than I'd intended. "I'll call as soon as I can," I added.

"O.K., O.K. Just let us know how you're doing."

I placed the receiver in its cradle, staving off tears that threatened to well up from my chest. I couldn't be homesick, I thought. I'd never been homesick in my life. But all my prior trips had come packaged with a return date. For the first time, home seemed impossibly far away. I ducked under the spider web that stretched across the doorway—the real reason I didn't want to use this pay phone again. I had zero desire to cross paths with the creator of such a menacing trap. My hand rose to my stomach before I realized that a dull ache had settled there.

I walked across the parking lot toward my room, stopping short when I noticed the immense mountains that framed the hotel in scenic backdrop. It looked like a movie set. I wondered how I could have missed that view before. The weather in Utah surpassed anything I'd experienced in central Pennsylvania. The views transcended breathtaking. How could I be anything but enraptured by it all? I gazed at the mountains for another moment. Then I went inside to watch more tennis.

15

TRANSFORMING THE NOW VACANT trailer into our new home felt like trying to complete someone else's half finished painting. The entire interior ensemble reminded me of the Vista Cruiser we'd had when I was a little girl. Same color scheme. Same wood paneling. The kitchen's color palette, including appliances, reflected varying shades of vomit, and the dark, faux wood walls throughout the trailer would require many gallons of white paint. We loaded up on tools and supplies to begin the weeklong process.

Before painting, Nick ripped out the desks that were built in to the corners of both extra bedrooms. We planned to turn those bedrooms into our offices and would replace the desks with slightly higher quality, assembly-required particleboard versions we'd purchased at Wal-Mart.

He showed me where to lay the plastic, so we didn't drip paint on the carpets, and how to tape off the areas we didn't want to paint. He poured the proper amount of paint into a shallow aluminum pan, loaded my roller with paint, then demonstrated how to roll it onto the walls.

"It's easy," he said. "You try." I took the roller from his hand and rolled it onto the wall, feeling an immediate sense of accomplishment as I watched the light spread to cover the dark.

"This is fun!" I said, and he laughed.

"Keep on having fun," he said. "I'm going to get started in the offices."

Nick hadn't asked for permission to redesign Rose's rental unit, which, in hindsight, should not have surprised me. He never told me how he smoothed the situation over after she learned of our remodeling frenzy. Perhaps she recognized some value in our efforts.

We opened up space in the bedrooms by removing those flimsy, built-in desks. Based on the fecal clues we found in doing so, it looked as if extended families of rodents had resided there. Our painting overhaul gave the trailer the lift we'd intended. With white, rather than brown-paneled walls, it felt lighter, more spacious, and more like the homes we were used to.

There was not much we could do about the puke-colored kitchen appliances. My mother would later explain to me that the proper term for the color was "harvest gold." Though Nick would have to enlist the help of more powerful friends than I to reinforce the river rock corner that was sinking beneath the woodburner, for now we could move our belongings out of the Quonset hut and into our new home.

I smiled at Nick and reached for his hand as we walked through the empty rooms surveying our handiwork. The kitchen was positioned at the end of the mobile home closest to Stringtown Road and opened, beyond the river rock half wall, into the living room. Off the hallway past the living room was an office for each of us, along with one full bath, which would easily suffice for two. The master bedroom sat at the end of the narrow hall. There was even a deck outside the back door that led to a fenced-in yard on the left and a one-and-a-half-car- or one-huge-truck-sized garage on the right. Nick would use that garage as his work area.

"Well," he said, "as far as solid constructions go, this place isn't winning any awards."

"But we did it." I turned to face him until he looked at me. I grabbed both of his hands and squeezed. "We have a house to live in!" He laughed and pulled me toward him.

"We did it," he said, holding me close for a moment. Then he pulled away and started toward the door, still holding on to my hand. "Now let's go get our furniture!"

Later that night, we curled up together on the futon couch and watched A Bug's Life on Nick's new PowerBook. I gazed across the room at the unpacked boxes and thought about what we'd accomplished so far. This was the start of our future. It may not seem like much now, but it was a foundation. I nestled against him and rested my head on his shoulder. From here, the doors of possibility were wide open.

The next morning, I sat in the living room unpacking boxes while Nick prepared to assemble our new desks. Katy and Chief sprawled out on the carpet, occasionally lifting their heads and sighing at the overall lack of action. They both jumped up when Rose knocked at the door. I braced myself for a reprimand about one or more of the changes we'd made as she stepped into the room, surveying our handiwork.

"Someone named Sue called my house for you," she said, and I nearly dropped the candlestick I'd been unwrapping.

"Do you know her?" I asked, trying to piece together how Sue could have found me.

"No, she must have called the campground. My friend in the office knew you were moving here."

"Oh!" I said. "Did she say what she wanted?" I was afraid to think what I wanted to think.

"She said she wants to offer you a job. You can come over to my house and use the phone." Rose smiled, and I stood to follow her. "The place looks nice," said over her shoulder to Nick as we walked out the door. I glanced back at him with saucer-wide eyes. Standing in the middle of the mud-brown, shag-carpeted living room surrounded by the assorted nuts, bolts, and flake board components of two identical, assembly-in-process computer desks, he cracked up laughing.

I started my job the very next week only to discover how hopelessly much I had to learn. Months later, Sue admitted that she'd hired me because she liked my personality. She'd worked with too many arrogant designers, and her number one requirement for the person filling this position was humility. As a homeless person desperate for a job, humility was my highest qualification. Though Sue had enough experience with graphic designers to know that I did not have enough experience for the job, she could tell my work ethic was solid, and my design skills had potential based on the portfolio pieces she'd seen. The expertise would come with experience, she'd wagered. If personality posed the problem, less manageable issues tended to ensue. This philosophy made perfect sense to me. I loved my new job. I earned almost double what I'd made in Pennsylvania, and Park City was glamorous.

I'd wake and shower each day at 6:00 a.m., then sit at the kitchen table and stare out the window toward the kennel as I ate my granola and milk. One time I watched a horse trot down the road with no saddle or harness or human in sight. Another time I emerged from the shower and glanced in the mirror over the sink to notice something in the reflection above my head. When I looked up, my heart nearly froze. Hanging from the ceiling three inches from my scalp was a glistening red spider the size of a plump grape. Its dagger-shaped legs, along with what looked to me like venomous fangs, pointed straight at my head. I ran to get Nick, who was sound asleep at 6:30 in the morning.

"Nick, wake up!" He didn't budge. "Nick, there's a really scary spider in the bathroom!" He groaned and rolled over. "Please!"

"What?"

"There's a spider!"

"Well get the jar..."

"No, it's poisonous."

"It isn't poisonous. Jesus, I was asleep." He grumbled the whole way to the spider jar in the kitchen then back to the bathroom where I directed him to the front of the mirror, and he stopped short. He stared at the spider in silence for a full thirty seconds.

"Get it!" I yelled. He jumped.

"O.K., O.K.," he said, milder now as he carefully positioned the jar under the monster. I couldn't watch.

Later that day, Sue took me to my first open house, where I had to resurrect some latent acting skills to hide my child-like wonder. The houses handled by my new employer reflected the colossal mountains that surrounded them. Encompassing upwards of 8,000 square feet, these cavernous homes boasted sky-scraping ceilings, sunken wet bars, solid marble floors and backsplashes, eight-burner ranges, refrigerators and cellars just for wine, distressed wood everything, outdoor fireplaces on wraparound decks, and heated garages and driveways, to name a few of the typical "amenities." I'd never even heard of a great room before and found myself so far outside of my architectural comfort zone that the only small talk I could conjure during that first open house revolved around the Godzilla-sized spider that had almost attacked my head that morning. I was new to the area. I had every reason to ask the natives if such an event represented the norm and what else I should prepare myself to expect from the local fauna and flora.

"Oh my god," said the woman I'd questioned. "If I were you, I'd bomb the shit out of my house."

"Really? Why?"

"It was probably a hobo or a brown recluse. You might have an infestation. Those things can kill you, or at least eat away your skin. I wouldn't mess around with that."

Eat away your skin? I couldn't very well tell the woman who was selling the million-plus-dollar home that I lived in an uninsulated trailer under which I was sure lived an unthinkable variety of creepy crawlies, poisonous and/or otherwise; that there would be no point in bombing my house-sized cardboard shoe box because nothing would prevent new monsters from crawling leisurely in as they pleased; that heaven knew what else was already planning its invasion as we spoke.

"Tara, you should try this chipotle chicken," Sue called from across the room, and a wave of nausea surged through me. The woman I'd been speaking to advised me to shake out my sweaters before putting them on because poisonous spiders liked to hide in sweaters. She put the fear of death and flesh-eating venom in me that day, and I never even got her name.

Nick later admitted that the spider had looked poisonous. "I wasn't about to tell *you* that!" he said.

Dan and Kelli thought it was probably a cat-face—the kind that looks poisonous but isn't. They'd seen those in the trailer before, they said, but never the really poisonous kind. This eased my mind by a fraction, but it would not stop me from shaking out my sweaters, banging my shoes upside down, and obsessively peeking under blankets, pillows, and bed sheets in search of monsters every day, probably for the rest of my life.

While I acclimated to my new job, Nick worked on acquiring the permits and licenses necessary to begin his mushing business. He launched a search to secure a veterinarian for the anticipated sled dogs in his future kennel. The only one who consented (but not, I later learned, without significant pleading on Nick's part) was a large animal vet—the same one who cared for Bart the Bear of *Legends of the Fall* and, among other movies, *The Bear*.

In November, he learned of a dog musher in Idaho who wanted to sell some of his sled dogs before going away to college. We hopped in the Jeep one Saturday morning and headed north toward Idaho to see what the musher had to offer. My previous experience with kennels had been with those that specialize in housing pets whose owners have gone on vacation. Katy had frequented several, and the ones I'd seen typically provided an enclosed dog run featuring both indoor and outdoor components for each canine resident. Loose within their respective runs, the dogs could wander in and out at their own discretion, depending on weather, nature's calling, curiosity, or boredom. Some kennels featured an open courtyard for supervised playtime.

The sled-dog kennel in Idaho bore little resemblance to the kennels of my memory. The indoor-outdoor accommodations here consisted of six-foot chains and rickety plywood boxes only slightly larger than the dogs themselves. Part of the kennel had been partitioned off with chicken wire, giving the whole assembly a shabby and ill-constructed appearance. Nick's kennel would be much more elegant, I knew, noticing at the same time that, despite my assessment of their accommodations, these dogs seemed not only healthy but happy. They jumped for joy when their owner led us into the chicken-wire enclosure, and the young musher gushed over them before pointing out the few he was willing to part with. All were close to six years old, and one could be used as a leader.

I left the kennel and walked back to the truck as Nick finished his negotiations, purchasing three dogs and bartering for one more—a two-year-old—in the process. By the end of the exchange, he walked away smiling, up four solid sled dogs for around six hundred dollars.

I had no point of reference for the monetary worth of a sled dog, but Nick was clearly pleased with his purchase. He loaded the dogs into the individual compartments he'd constructed within the plywood box for this specific purpose. As we drove away, the young musher held up his hand in a single wave, and I thought I saw a tear in his eye.

We rode in silence as I thought about the events of the day. I'd just taken part in the bartering of living creatures.

"Are you sure they're O.K. back there?" I asked. I hadn't noticed how tiny the compartments looked before watching Nick hoist the dogs into them. Each dog had turned around so that its nose pressed against the slatted window, but I couldn't stop wondering if those slats allowed enough airflow for comfort.

"They're fine," Nick said. "This is how it's done." I stifled the rest of my questions. Whether or not I would ever learn more about Nick's chosen line of work, I had to trust now that he knew what he was doing.

Among Nick's new sled dogs was Jax, an eight-year-old male with a short, white coat, tinged with gray down his back, and pale blue eyes. He was stoic and standoffish with strangers. The other male was Rocky, built like a horse and pure white except for the black mask that covered his eyes and ears. At two-years old, Rocky acted like a teenage boy. Edie was an Australian Shepherd mix, spring-loaded with energy and taut with solid muscle. And Whisky—the new matriarch—was a six-year old sound leader of a dog with a full coat of silver and black framing the lighter gray whiskers of her muzzle. Whisky's wide, amber eyes searched for constant approval.

These and other sled dogs would play a formative role in my life over the next two years, but I didn't know that as I sat in the warm Jeep thinking about the four transients tucked away in the straw-filled wooden boxes behind us. Did they wonder where we were taking them? Had they been through this process enough times in their lives that they no longer bothered to wonder?

16

PARK CITY WAS A WONDERLAND that came alive at winter's peak. An outsider like myself might initially equate the term "fresh powder" with "bomb scare" based on the speed and efficiency with which sixty plus real estate agents cleared the building when word of "fresh powder" reached them. It happened often, and it never failed to surprise me. As a native easterner, the concept of abandoning work for fun in the middle of the day completely escaped me (an attitude which proved convenient, since it wasn't an option for the administrative staff, including me, who were salaried to adhere to a more traditional 8:00 to 5:00 schedule). The behavior didn't seem natural and neither did the weather conditions that positively reinforced it.

In central Pennsylvania, the sun began its hibernation as early as October. A blanket of cloud cover grayed out the sky for so many months in a row that by the time the sun returned in spring, you'd almost forgotten it ever existed. But here in Park City, sunshine dominated the sky upwards of 225 days per year. It must have been a result of the ample sunshine that people never seemed downtrodden or melancholy, I thought. That or the plastic surgery I'd recently heard was all the rage in the area. One thing I knew. Park City sparkled in winter like a manmade diamond—just a little too flawless to feel completely authentic.

Park City's positive energy during the holiday season did nothing to improve the attitude Nick and I shared about spending Christmas in Utah. We were homesick, and we were stuck. I hadn't yet earned vacation time at my new job, and Nick had the sled dogs to feed and water every day. For the first time in my life, I would miss spending Christmas with my family.

It was time to grow up, I told myself every time the thought of spending Christmas away from home pulled me into a whirlpool of nostalgia. I tried to redirect my mind toward the positive possibilities; this would be a new adventure, as would Thanksgiving, for which I harbored a different attitude altogether.

For our family Thanksgiving dinner, my mother always opted for the basic staples of turkey, stuffing, cranberry sauce, and corn. Such traditional Thanksgiving fare bored my taste buds to apathy, and I looked forward to experimenting with some new recipes for the meal I would cook in Utah. I was inclined to skip the turkey altogether, but the nostalgia whirlpool intervened. Without the turkey, I couldn't be certain the food I prepared would qualify as a Thanksgiving meal.

My attempt to maintain that element of tradition failed. When the pop-up timer hadn't popped up from our less-than-ten-pound turkey after more than four hours in the oven, it dawned on us that some pop-up timers were probably defective. It was, of course, too late. Our Thanksgiving turkey was reduced to the approximate consistency of wood shavings after a light drizzle. The flavor, I had to presume, was only marginally better. It wasn't a total loss. As I'd focused my efforts on redesigning side dishes, skimping on the less-than-palatable turkey freed up tummy space for those new creations.

I'd replaced the traditional corn and pea combination of my brother's liking with a baked creamed corn recipe Grammie had provided over the phone that week. Rather than wrapping the yams in foil, like my mother always did, I threw them, peeled and chopped, into a casserole dish and doused them with melted butter and brown sugar before baking. I went out on an experimental limb with a new recipe of baked asparagus with mushrooms and artichoke hearts, and I whipped the red potatoes, skins on, with a stick of salted butter and a generous dose of heavy cream. Nick prepared a bread stuffing, which, in my side-dish cooking extravaganza, I'd decided not to bother with. We heated crusty French rolls, slathered them with soft butter, and cracked open a bottle of chardonnay for our Thanksgiving in Utah. There were two of us, and we'd made enough food for a family of eight.

As a general rule Nick didn't eat much, but I hailed from a family of overachievers in that department. Years of practice had helped me to perfect the art. During college, food money was scarce, and I typically spent the little I did have on beer. My nutritional survival strategy involved fasting during the week then showing up at Grammie's apartment on Sunday evening in hopes of finding something home-cooked and binge-worthy awaiting my voracious consumption. The tactic never failed. Grammie would smile as I curled up in her plush La-Z-Boy recliner to relish my chicken soup with vegetables and dumplings, or my pounded steak with gravy, or whatever home-cooked meal she'd happened to have the ingredients to throw together during my not-so-surprise visit. She knew it was going to be the only decent meal I would eat all week.

Over the years I'd morphed into one of those annoying people who can eat three times their body weight in any food group of their choosing while gaining no weight to speak of. I still hadn't put on the ten pounds I'd lost before moving to Utah. I did often suffer the pain and bloating of my overeating tendencies, but I'd grown to accept that small payment in stride. The effects were uncomfortable but tolerable, and I secretly loved the fact that I could eat like a grizzly bear preparing for hibernation and not gain any weight in the process. That Thanksgiving, Nick and I avoided the loneliness of our isolation from family and friends by filling ourselves up with food. It worked out well enough, but Christmas was another story.

Shortly after Thanksgiving, Nick picked up a Christmas tree at the local hardware store. It was a simple, artificial tree that took no effort to erect—small and thin and a little bit sad. We fell in love with it. We strung a few colored lights and hung one or two ornaments, which were all the little tree could bear on its pipe cleaner limbs.

We sat next to our tree on the dirt-colored rug in the living room and drank coffee on chilled December mornings, soaking in warmth from the woodburning stove. Every few minutes, a sound akin to gunfire emanated from that stove to jolt us alert. The popping noises resulted from exploding sap in the piñon wood we bought to burn. The chimney would get so hot it would glow bright orange. One time it actually exploded. I was standing in the living room about six feet away from the stove when the elbow joint burst away from the middle of the chimney, and billows of black smoke poured into the living room. Nick was in the shower but not for long after my shrieking started. Clad in only a bath towel, he grabbed some oven mitts and carefully lodged the critical joint back into position while I opened the front and back doors to make a wind tunnel for the smoke to escape. That was life in our little Midway trailer home. We never knew what to expect next.

In Park City, Christmastime triggered a level of glee—an almost contagious ecstasy—that would normally peck away at my patience. But a couple of days before Christmas, the agents started delivering gifts to my cubicle. Sue explained this phenomenon as the agents' way of thanking the administrative staff for all our hard work that year. We admins, she assured me, were not expected to reciprocate.

By the time Christmas Eve rolled around, I had more presents from those real estate agents than I usually received from my own family. I brought all those gifts home, fully wrapped, and placed them under our Charlie Brown tree. When I woke up Christmas morning and walked out to the living room, Nick was sitting beside that woodburning stove holding a mug of coffee and staring at all the presents. He wore his usual plaid flannel top and fleece pajama bottoms. His feet were bare, and his hair stood wildly on end. I laughed and shook my head.

"Where are your slippers?" I said. "It's freezing in here."

He looked up at me and grinned. "Let's open presents!"

We started with presents from the real estate agents, followed by those our families had sent in the mail. Katy had opened her own presents from the very first Christmas after I'd brought her home, without any coaxing at all. She'd choose the package meant for her among all the others under the tree. Then she'd lie down and unwrap it, gently pulling the paper off in strips by using her front teeth to catch and tear, then shaking her head to discard the torn paper before starting on another strip. In this manner, she uncovered an orange and purple sock toy that my parents had lovingly sent and that Chief immediately confiscated.

"Time for ours," I said. "You first." I handed Nick his present.

"It's small," he said, holding it up to his ear.

"You can't hear it," I laughed. "Just open it." He tore the paper away and opened the box to reveal a sterling silver Native American cuff bracelet.

"Wow, sweetie, this is great. Where did you get this?"

"In Park City. I saw you looking at them when we were shopping. You seemed to like the Hopi designs best."

"I do, I really like the silver and black together. Thank you," he said putting the bracelet on and leaning over to kiss my cheek. "I feel bad now. My present for you isn't this nice."

"I'm sure it's fine," I said, tearing the paper to reveal a jumbo white plastic digital alarm clock radio. "What the..."

"I know, it isn't good," he laughed. "I just thought it would help you wake up in the morning."

"I wake up in the morning." I said, still staring at the box in my hand.

"Well that antique bell alarm you have is terrifying. I almost piss myself every time it goes off, and you reset it three times every morning."

"I'm just trying not to be late," I said.

"If you really cared, the alarm clock wouldn't have anything to do with it." I tore my eyes away from the clock and looked at Nick.

"What are you talking about?"

"Just that you shouldn't be late all the time," he said, and I paused as his meaning settled in.

"Nick, that's just the way I am. I'm not trying to be late, and you know," I said, thinking more clearly, "my family and friends always accepted this about me."

"Tara, when you're late, you're telling people their time isn't as important as yours." My mouth opened, but no sound came out. I looked down at my new plastic clock.

"Let's just drop it," Nick said. "I thought you could use a new clock, so I got you one. It's a lame present." He smiled. "Hey, why don't I put on some Bing Crosby. Or Sinatra. Nobody can resist Sinatra singing Christmas carols." He bent his head toward me until I was forced to look at his goofy smile. *"Haaaave yoooooouurself a merry little Christmaaaas,"* he crooned. I shoved the alarm clock into his lap.

"Jerk," I said. Nick smiled wider and touched my cheek. "Do you really almost pee in your pants every time my alarm goes off?" I asked, and he laughed. Then he stood up to put on some Christmas CDs.

We finished our coffee by the dimly lit tree, listening to music and examining our gifts. Later that afternoon, we opened the front door to find that someone had left an orange on our doorstep. *How nice,* I thought, transported for the moment to a familiar place in the old fashioned kitchen of my grammie's house, years before she moved into an apartment. She would cut an orange in half and go to work on carving out the wedges between the rinds with her knife. Then she'd sprinkle heaping teaspoons of sugar on top of each half. I'd watch the sugar turn from white to translucent as it dissolved into the orange. Grammie would spoon the wedges, one at a time, into my mouth as I stood on my tippytoes over the double-basin porcelain sink, craning my neck to reach each syrupy bite. When we were all finished with the orange wedges, she would cut another orange down the middle and twist each half onto the glass juicer. She'd pour the juice through the strainer that sat on top of my glass, then she'd squeeze two drops of her diabetic sweetener into the juice, stirring it in before she handed it to me. The extra sweetness of the first sip always stayed in my mouth even after I swallowed. That Christmas in Utah, I could almost taste the extra sweetness of Grammie's oranges on my tongue as I picked up the orange on our doorstep, briefly wondering who had left it there and why.

Later that day, I cooked chicken divan, white rice, tossed salad, and garlic bread—my family's traditional Christmas meal since before I was born. Nick and I each talked on the phone to our parents, and they passed the phone around for us to say hello to everyone else who was there. My mother, my father, my grammie, my brother. Nick's sister, his mother, his nephew. We were all celebrating, having our own separate feasts, but this time in Utah, the feasting didn't succeed in filling us up. I felt like all the food in the world couldn't have filled me up that Christmas, and I made the decision right then and there never to spend another Christmas away from home. Nick did not hesitate to agree.

17

WHILE I FOCUSED ON MY job in Park City, Nick searched for dogs to fill the kennel and collaboration opportunities for touring locations and clientele. During that time, he used his web skills to build an income-generating business. He'd learned how to make sure his mother's website showed up in popular search engines—"ranking," he called it. Now, he offered that service to larger companies. This burgeoning "e-commerce" business of Nick's set my mind at ease. Reputable companies would surely pay for this valuable service, I thought, allowing Nick to phase out the "adult" business element on which he'd previously had to rely. In the coming months, he would cultivate his knowledge and skills by collaborating virtually with a network of peers and attending conferences across the globe. This Internet expertise of Nick's, as far as I could tell, financially sustained his portion of our domestic life in Utah, along with the rest of his dog mushing dream.

We shared all household expenses—from electric bills and rent to the cost of necessities like groceries, firewood, and beer—as equally as possible. Neither of us worried about how much money the other made, saved, or spent as long as we produced our rent and beer money. I suspected Nick sometimes borrowed from his father, but just as his earnings never impacted my own financial status, neither did his debt. The situation was mutual, and maintaining our individuality in this area conformed to a philosophy my mother had bestowed upon me from the time I was a little girl. "You have to make your own money," she'd say when the subject of financial independence arose and, "Don't ever rely on a man to take care of you." (She sometimes proclaimed that I'd better marry a rich man to support my expensive tastes, but I sensed a lack of conviction in that advice.)

During my busiest months at work, I thought about renting an apartment in Park City to be closer to my job, but Nick squelched the idea seconds after I uttered it. "My dad likes his girlfriends on the side," he said, and, though I failed to fully comprehend the connection, I understood that he did not approve.

Disparities between Nick and his father were nuggets of hope I latched onto, and I found notably fewer as time passed. I saw in Nick an eclectic genetic combination of his father, the self-made millionaire, and his mother, the struggling artist who, I also learned, was bipolar. Nick's mother was the most talented artist I'd ever met, and I wondered if talent like that always came at a price. Though I barely knew her, I credited Nick's mother for the qualities I most admired in Nick—his creativity and appreciation for art, his kindness and respect for nature, and his frequent words of wisdom. Now I learned that this dog-mushing dreamer I'd followed out west had every intention of becoming a millionaire, just like his father. He would not accomplish this through dog mushing, I realized. In addition to the cost of purchasing dogs, Nick poured an endless stream of money into food and vet bills, not to mention mushing equipment and kennel provisions. But as long as the dogs were happy and healthy, it didn't much matter to me what else Nick chose to do with his money or, for that matter, how exactly he earned it. Perhaps it should have.

Nick planned to connect with a ski resort in Park City or Salt Lake City to run his dog sled tours. Ski resorts in those areas had plenty of extra land, not to mention snow, for dog sled trails, and they drew an abundance of customers from October through March. These customers, Nick thought, would likely enjoy an alternative sporting activity to skiing, and the resorts could benefit financially from diversifying.

He called and visited resorts to discuss the options for offering this distinctive opportunity to future clients. If the price was right, he might even agree to partner, making one resort the exclusive provider of authentic dog sled tours in the greater Park City or Salt Lake City area. One by one, each resort turned him down. Due to prohibitive business laws or liability fears or basic lack of interest—for whatever reasons—not a single resort came to agreeable terms.

Nick directed his focus closer to home, inquiring about Soldier Hollow—the site just down the road that had been slated as the 2002 Olympic biathlon venue—but he ran into complications there, too. He'd sometimes grumble about Utah's "weird" business laws, but I never grasped many of the details. Winter months were notoriously busy at the real estate company, and I was beginning to buckle under the demands of my limited design experience.

While Nick worked on his various businesses, I buried myself in creating real estate ads, newsletters, flyers, and the full-sized magazine that the company published every year around the time of the Sundance Film Festival. This glorified real estate booklet featured separate sections to highlight the geographic areas in which homes and commercial properties were available for purchase. It also prevailed as the pride of the company owner—his annual chance to showcase his company and accomplishments in one glossy booklet. Sue hired the most elite professional photographers, worked hand-in-hand with an exclusive printer in Salt Lake City, and chose the finest inks to decorate the glossiest pages to showcase the zillion-dollar behemoths that people built and bought as vacation homes. The company spared no expense. I presumed that a company specializing in the sale of homes whose values often ranged upwards of several million dollars had no reason to spare an expense, but Sue had more knowledge than I in that area. I should have known I was in over my head when I saw the quality of the previous year's edition, or when Sue hired a professional artist to grace the cover with an original illustration, or when she told me it was costing $20,000—more than half of my salary—to produce that booklet.

Instead of triggering an alert beacon about my own abilities, the cost of that magazine fed my already inflated perception of the job's importance and the glam factor of Park City, in general. The moment I thought I'd experienced all there was to adore about Park City, the Sundance Film Festival rolled into town, and celebrities swarmed along with it like locusts. Sightings were popping up everywhere. I struggled to suppress my desire, but the thought of spotting a real-live celebrity captivated me. I knew my chance had come. Working in the heart of Park City during the Sundance Film Festival set me up for a sure sighting. It didn't matter that most native Utahans avoided Park City during film festival week in the same way they might avoid a seeping vat of infectious waste. I planned to enter the celebrity pool discreetly rather than diving in head first. I wouldn't dress in black, for example. I would simply stroll up and down Main Street over the lunch hour looking like the Park City real estate company graphic designer I was, just out for a quick bite on my lunch break. At least some celebrities probably went to lunch, I reasoned, whether or not they ate actual food.

When Sue returned from an appointment one afternoon and told me she'd seen Kevin Spacey crossing Main Street, I made my celebrity-spotting aspirations clear.

"I've never seen a celebrity in real life," I said in admiration of her accomplishment.

"Well don't go into town now. It's a madhouse." She must have misinterpreted my point. One of the agent's assistants drifted into our cubicle to drop off a proof. "I just saw Kevin Spacey on Main Street," Sue said.

"Oh yeah?" The assistant seemed unimpressed. "I saw Frances McDormand at lunch yesterday."

"Wow," I said, "I've never seen a celebrity."

"Oh, I see them all the time," said the assistant. "I'm like a celebrity magnet." Then she floated away before I could learn more about this intriguing quality.

Adverse to my celebrity-spotting plans, the annual magazine super-glued me to my desk from just past dawn to well after dusk every day that week. I never even left the office to eat lunch, let alone to catch a glimpse of a celebrity. Weeks later, when I did have time to join Sue for lunch at a restaurant on Main Street, she would point out Victoria Principal, sitting in a corner booth. When she walked by our table to leave, I made an effort to stare, but I could not discern the quality for which I searched—the one that separates celebrities into such an elite and privilege-deserving group. This star quality was so clear in movies and magazines and on TV. I was sure it would be visible in the flesh. *I must be missing something*, I thought, as I watched the pretty, miniscule figure walk out the door and disappear down the street.

As the number of my daily and weekly office hours increased with the production of the annual magazine, I struggled to process the tsunami of new information required to perform all the functions of my job. If I had my suspicions of underperforming, Sue never confirmed them. Not a scowl or a word of disappointment spouted from Sue, who brimmed only with encouragement and sound advice.

Sue's guidance saved me from a torrent of ignorance-driven humiliations, not the least of which related to a print industry concept I'd been unable to assimilate. For weeks I racked my brain for a clue as to what post-menstrual syndrome had to do with a printing press. I was on the verge of hatching my own theory on the temperamental nature of the business or of the presses themselves when Sue discreetly informed me that PMS referred to the Pantone Matching System (PMS) of colors used by the printing industry. She also pointed out that a "four-color print job" was another way of saying a full-color print job because in offset printing, only four colors—cyan, magenta, yellow, and black (aka CMYK)—combined to produce full-color pieces like photographic images. "Two colors" really meant two colors, I was relieved to discover, and "three colors" was an option used only by show-offs.

The advice Sue dispensed transcended print design wisdom. She saw me turning to the vending machine for pretzels on a regular basis in attempt to assuage my frequent stomachaches. Noticing that my self-induced remedy failed every time, Sue recommended an alternative that sounded so ridiculous I couldn't convince myself to try it. In search of a consumable product bland enough to relieve my tumultuous digestive system, I thought, pretzels represented the only logical choice. This thought pattern persisted, and my stomachaches worsened until relentless discomfort forced logic's surrender. I tried Sue's suggestion of Coca-Cola, and almost magically, it worked.

I learned more from Sue than from any boss I'd ever had or any that were yet to come. She connected me with the right printers, photographers, and designers to build my skills and learn the craft of graphic design through experience and, I can't deny it, trial by fire. I didn't get it all right, but the portfolio I built during the time I worked under Sue would carry me through many more years of position shifts in the graphic design industry. As a mentor and boss, Sue was creative and socially gifted but not necessarily detail oriented. Project management was not Sue's primary strength. Unfortunately, it wasn't mine either. When the time came in December to create the magazine in digital format, I found myself, three days before deadline, with sixty-four pages worth of loose photographs and hand-written notes. I worked the greater part of the next seventy-two hours to make deadline on that magazine. By the time I finished, an affliction beyond exhaustion besieged my body. My head throbbed and my chest ached, and I holed up in bed for three full days.

Two weeks later, after most of the magazines had been distributed, I learned that the image we'd used in the first section of the magazine—a professional photograph taken from the bottom of the hill looking straight up Park City's Main Street—was reversed. The slide had been scanned upside-down, and our $20,000 magazine now showcased Park City's prestigious Main Street shops on the opposite sides of reality. The company owner avoided my presence. The vice president said I looked "green around the gills." Sue spoke not one word on the subject. Soon after that, she told me her husband had taken a job in Colorado and she'd be moving in the next several weeks. After four months with the company, my foundation was already cracking.

18

ON ONE OF MY WEEKEND KENNEL visits, I asked why each of the sled dogs looked so different. There were similarities in build and personality, but Nick's kennel had everything from jet-black, short-haired dogs to almost pure-white, thick-coated dogs of varying weights and sizes.

"They're Alaskan huskies," he told me. "They can be a mix of different breeds."

"I thought sled dogs were Siberian huskies," I said, noting that Rocky's mask looked like nothing I'd ever seen on a Siberian.

"Some people run straight Siberians," Nick said, "but most run Alaskans. They're faster for racing."

"I used to watch dog shows with my dad sometimes," I said, following Nick as he traversed the kennel, stopping every few feet to scoop poop with his pointed-nose garden shovel. "I wonder why I've never heard of an Alaskan husky?"

"They aren't recognized as a breed by the AKC," Nick said as he dumped a shovel load into a plastic, five-gallon bucket. "Alaskans can be a combination of just about anything—usually a northern breed like Siberians or malamutes, because they're accustomed to colder climates, and maybe greyhounds for speed. Some people even breed hound dogs into the mix for better endurance."

"Do people still use sled dogs for anything other than sport?" I asked.

"There are still lots of working dogs in Alaska and probably in other northern places," he said.

Thinking of the dog shows I'd seen on TV, it seemed to me there should have been a way to determine the perfect genetic blend for sled dogs, just like there had been for all those other breeds. The distinction, I supposed, lay in their canine careers. For all I knew, many show dogs had never been exposed to a profession other than that of parading around the ring as the perfect physical examples of their breeds. The supermodels of the canine world, I thought. Scanning the kennel full of Alaskan huskies that day, I found myself wondering if those show dogs would have enjoyed a more genetically relevant profession.

Fairly new to the kennel was Lancelot, a striking male who, of all the dogs, most resembled a Siberian husky. Lancelot lacked a comparable brain to balance his brawn. When he urinated, he walked in tight circles, alternately lifting and dropping each hind leg while turning, mid-stream, in three-legged hops and peeing all over himself every ill-fated time. Stale urine permeated Lancelot from the undercoat out, resulting in extreme effort on my part to avoid all contact without protective gear like Carhartt coveralls and all-weatherproof gloves. If developmental disorders were assigned to canines, Lancelot would have been the ADHD poster puppy. I believed this quality endeared him to Nick. I also believed Nick had saved that dog's life.

The day he brought Lancelot home, Nick called me out to the back deck.

"Look at this," he said, parting the hair on the dog's neck.

"Oh my god." The stench of rotting skin drifted toward me, and I raised my hand to my mouth. "Is that his collar?" I bent down, my hand now covering my nose, and I squinted to determine where the collar ended and Lancelot's skin began. The two seemed fused together.

"It's infected," Nick said. "I've got to get that collar off."

Lancelot lived collar-free in the fenced-in backyard until he was well enough to move into the kennel with the rest of the sled dogs. Nick cleaned his wounds and applied antibiotics several times a day during that time, talking to him gently and forming a special bond with his future team member. Each time I visited the kennel after Lancelot's recovery, I was sure to see Nick fawning all over that beautiful, stinky dog. And Lancelot clung to Nick's side, in turn.

Nick had purchased a pair of sisters at the same time he purchased Lancelot. Each weighed less than forty pounds, which Nick said was small for sled dogs. Snowball was a female wad of energy with a coat of cotton breached only by searching brown eyes and a soft pink nose. I suspected Snowball might forego a drink of water after a forty-mile run if it brought her an extra moment of human affection. Her sister, Cinnamon, a reddish-spice-shaded beauty with eyes of flecked gold, was a fraction less needy than her sister. This she made up for in spunk. Nick had been training the dogs by taking small teams out to run together a couple of times a week, but my frantic work schedule had prevented my joining him for a ride. I still couldn't grasp the concept of dogs pulling a sled behind them just for the sake of it.

"They love to run," Nick often assured me.

"But why?" I inevitably replied.

"That's what they're bred to do," he said every time. "It's in their blood."

This line of reasoning felt incomplete. It seemed futile to ask if those dogs would pull a sled minus the human-directed training they'd received since birth, conditioning them to do so. *I'd love to run too*, I refrained from verbalizing, *if I spent most of my life tethered to a six-foot chain.*

On most days, Nick let the dogs run loose in the kennel for a couple hours of exercise and team building. My firsthand lesson in the canine world of team building came on an otherwise typical Sunday afternoon during one of my kennel visits. By that time, a total of nine dogs comprised Nick's kennel, which he'd decided to call SnowDog Racing & Touring in hopes of someday securing all the necessary legal agreements and finding a location to run tours. I had walked across the road toward the fenced-in area of the barnyard that Nick had fashioned into the kennel. I was almost to the entrance when he spotted me. He saw that I'd brought beer, smiled, then started toward the oversized metal gate that served as the kennel door. The dogs followed closely behind and, as Nick and I hoisted the rusted gate using our combined weights, all nine dogs converged at the opening. Nick blocked the opening with his body, pushing the eager dogs' noses back from the crack.

"Pull it closed," he said. "We'll try again in a minute." When all the dogs were loose, I rarely made it into the kennel on the first attempt. Sometimes we made three or four, each with close canine escape calls, before I succeeded. Today, as Nick and I focused on closing the gate, we heard a series of unusual barks that morphed into a pandemonium of vicious growls. We looked up to see all nine dogs engaged in a barbaric brawl. I stood frozen as the flashing pink gums of snarling, biting dogs blurred into a mass of fur, then the raging growls fell to sinister silence. *Was that Whisky in the middle?* I squinted, unable to believe what I thought I saw.

Nick plunged into the savage mix, forcing his way between dogs while grabbing and kicking to separate the huddle.

"Noooooo!" I screamed in helpless reaction while Nick, in a few short seconds, had pulled most of the dogs apart. My adrenaline surge found its delayed release, and I took off around the perimeter of the kennel calling all the names that came to my mind. "Whisky, Whisky, come on Whisky! Cinnamon! Snowball! Lancelot! Come on Lancey boy!" Some of the dogs noticed me and moved away from the scuffle, allowing Nick to chain the others to their stakes in rapid succession.

After securing the last dog, Nick surveyed the kennel then looked at me through the slats in the fence. In that split second of eye contact, a bubble of tension popped. We broke into nervous laughter, then sighed with relief at having so narrowly averted catastrophe. I walked back to the gate to let myself into the kennel and handed Nick a bottle of beer. After taking an extended swig, he made his way around to each dog and checked for battle wounds. To my surprise, he found none. The dogs had long since resumed their playful demeanor, looking somewhat confused at their current state of confinement. *What's the problem?* they seemed to be wondering, as if kennel brawls were a common occurrence. Then it dawned on me that they probably were. While this scuffle represented my first experience with the formation of canine hierarchies, the dogs, I realized, were innately familiar with this natural process. That was the day Whisky established herself as the formidable leader of the pack. And Nick, forever after, would be the alpha male.

I'd often contemplated the concept of equilibrium—wondering if some universal force drove the elements of nature toward a state of balance. Opposite forces in nature had a tendency to attract, I'd observed over the years, though true equilibrium seemed fleeting to the verge of impossible. Still, the idea of balance as a goal had always made sense to me. My experiences with the dogs sparked an ember of faith in this concept.

Months of living in the run-down mobile home had failed to acclimate me to the popping piñon in the woodburner, the sinking floor underneath that woodburner, or the whistling winds that sometimes pushed the battered old trailer to the brink of impending flight. These elements that threatened our world drew Nick and me closer. We were in this struggle together—the young couple starting a fresh new life. Things would get better, and our bond would be stronger for all that we'd gone through. We'd look back on these times with fond memories. The trailer was only a launching point.

But for all the frights, frustrations, and inconveniences of our makeshift living quarters, one paramount saving grace transcended anything built by human hands, and all Nick or I had to do to access that grace was walk outside. Across the street from our less-than-regal mobile home loomed a majestic wealth of wilderness. In addition to having unobstructed views of the second highest peak in Utah—Mount Timpanogos—we lived on the road that led to the Soldier Hollow Olympic venue. Between our trailer and Soldier Hollow was a right-hand turn that led to Cascade Springs, a popular attraction off the Alpine Loop Scenic Byway that we'd traversed so many times that fall. Cascade Springs road (as we had come to refer to it) was impassable in winter, and that made it a perfectly acceptable, though treacherously steep, sled dog training track.

The first time Nick took me on a dog sled ride I almost chickened out before he'd even hooked all the dogs up to the sled. It was ten o'clock at night. The moonlight radiated off the snow, illuminating the world around us in a mystical glow. I thought I'd seen everything after that rumble in the kennel. I'd soon discover I hadn't even come close.

Nick's handmade wooden racing sled was approximately six feet in length, crafted with long, slender strips of White Ash that Nick had glued and clamped to precise specifications before securing each with hand-tied knots of the strongest fishing line he could find. With a forward thrusting brush bow that mirrored the curve of the upright drive bow, this sled was as graceful as it was sleek. In the center of the sled, sitting delicately atop the six-foot long runners, was the basket—traditionally built to hold supplies, untraditionally built to hold me. Nick had lined the sled with thick blankets, topped with a sleeping bag, which he unzipped in preparation for our quick takeoff. He would drive, standing up at the back of the sled. I would ride, snug inside the blankets in the cargo basket.

Nick set the claw brake and, for extra security, dug the snow hook deep into the snow behind the sled before instructing me on how it was all going to happen. He would hook the two leaders up first, Whisky and Shane. I was to stand up front with them, holding the line between them and making sure they didn't get tangled as he hooked up the other dogs, one by one.

Got it, I thought, no problem. I took my position at the end of the lines, only then noticing how long the lines actually were. The lead dogs, by my estimation, would be a good twenty feet from the front of the sled. As I stood considering the implications of such long lines, Nick came running toward me with a frantic Whisky beside him. He had to hold her up by the chain so that her two front feet didn't touch the ground. Otherwise he would have had no chance of keeping a hold on this dog that was bred to run. Even with Nick's restraints, Whisky plunged forward on her hind legs in giant leaps, and I realized that if her two front feet were to make contact with the ground, that dog would be gone in a flash to anywhere. I was beginning to get nervous. Once Nick hooked Whisky up to the line, she surged forward in a frenzy, jerking the sled off its runners behind her.

"Hold her!" Nick yelled, and he raced back to get another dog. I tried my best to hold Whisky by the shoulders and convince her to contain her mania. Next came Shane, our gentle black giant whose only previous mission in life seemed to be that of sweetly pining for as much attention as he could get. I wasn't worried about Shane, until I saw the look in his wildly possessed eyes. The Shane Nick attached to the line next to Whisky seemed to be inhabited by the spirit of a dog I hadn't yet met—one that I probably wouldn't have cared to, given the opportunity for a choice. While Whisky had only partially accommodated my firm directive of settling down, Shane would have none of it. The sixty-pound wad of muscle lunged forward with all his might and from the depths of his throat came blood-curdling sounds that didn't seem natural. A cross between a howling bellow and an agonized wail launched with every thrusting lunge. The little wooden sled dangled on the end of the flailing lines, and my blankets went asunder in the jumble.

"HOLD HIM!" Nick shouted as he approached the next set of lines with Cinnamon. By that time, I was as frantic as the dogs were, yelling back at them and forcing my arms between the two leaders as they barked and screeched and yowled in my ears. The mind-numbing ruckus only amplified as more dogs took their places in line.

I have one job, I told myself, *to keep the leaders untangled and steady.* At one point, Cinnamon and Snowball appeared to have switched positions, and before I'd completed my double-take, Nick sprinted forward to untangle them. As I watched him fling little Cinnamon over the line and back into proper position, I saw Jax jump straight up in the air and land on Midnight. Both dogs started jumping, and lines twisted everywhere. Nick continued up and down the lines of dogs, fixing the tangles and adjusting positions. The dogs seemed determined to raise the dead with their heart-pumping uproar.

I have one job, I kept telling myself. My breath came in short gasps. My heart beat like a hummingbird's, ready to explode. *One job*, I thought.

"Come on, come on, get in the sled!" Nick shouted from the helm. I released my hold on Shane and broke into a run, jumping into the sled and falling clumsily into the cushion of blankets just as the hook came loose.

"HAaaaa-Ayyyyke!" Nick shouted.

Whoooshhhh! We were off like an arrow into the night, and absolute silence echoed in my ears.

Shhhhhhhh, Shhhhhhhhh, Shhhhhhhhh . . . Nick's delicate wooden sled glided over the snow like a ballerina on her stage.

"Wow," I whispered.

"Cover up," Nick said, reaching down to pull the sleeping bag around me. I adjusted my position after having fallen so haphazardly into the sled. I pulled my hat over my ears and nestled into the blankets, drinking in the silent beauty of the winter night. As the dogs slowed to pace, a light snow began to fall.

"What do you think?" Nick asked. He couldn't see the tears in my eyes.

"Unreal," I said.

The ride lasted for about an hour. We went part of the way up Cascade Springs road before turning around for the descent. It was a hairy turnaround in the middle of the night on a narrow pass, but by that time a kind of absurd tranquility had infiltrated my body, penetrating to the depths of my soul, and nothing short of launching over the side of that mountain was likely to shake me up again. The dogs seemed to have found their balance as well, never fidgeting or making a sound after the initial disarray. This was a team in harmony, I realized, not caring that I had no earthly idea as to how it had all come together.

This was why the goal of equilibrium made so much sense, I thought, remembering the initial chaos of the ride's onset. The absolute harmony of the ride outweighed the chaos of the preparation, and for a fleeting moment, I wondered how chaos would regain its ground in the never-ending struggle toward balance.

The next day I floated around the kitchen preparing our brunch, still mesmerized from the previous night's dog sledding experience. I fried some potatoes, toasted four slices of bread, and cooked our respective eggs—mine over-easy and Nick's sunny-side up, the way he liked them. We sat at the table in contented silence.

"Hey," I said, finally shattering our reverie as a memory from the dog sled ride popped into my head. "You never said mush."

"Huh?" Nick looked up from dipping his toast into the sunny part of his egg.

"Mush," I repeated. "You're supposed to say mush when you mush dogs. You never said it."

"Nobody says mush," he informed me. "The dogs wouldn't even know what to do. You may as well say banana," he smiled.

"What?" I couldn't believe it. "Then why is it called dog mushing?"

"I have no idea. I've never heard anyone say mush in all the years I've run dogs. The word is completely meaningless," Nick said, and he pushed his plate away, the whites of his eggs still completely intact with the indentation of a perfect round circle where the sun used to be.

PART III

The Life I Signed Myself Up For

19

SUE'S IMPENDING DEPARTURE put me in a generalized funk. The Saturday after I'd heard, I ventured across the street with Nick for a dose of sled-dog therapy. Being around the dogs while they raced and played and sometimes body slammed me in ebullient greeting had a way of lifting my spirits. But one glance at Midnight ensured I would not find solace in the dogs that day. His typically bright brown eyes had faded behind lead-filled lids, and his cone-shaped ears that always stood at attention, giving him the appearance of a jet-black Rin Tin Tin, now sagged off opposite sides of his head, as if gravity had grown too great a force for them to fight. I walked toward him.

"This dog is sick," I said to Nick.

"I know," Nick said. "He's been like that for a week. I'm taking him to the vet on Monday." Before I could crouch down, Midnight hoisted himself against me and wrapped his two front legs around my torso, mimicking his brother's signature bear hug in a display never before executed by him. He looked me in the eyes, then leaned his whole body into mine.

He's asking me to do something, I thought. I rubbed Midnight's ears and told him everything was going to be O.K. "We'll get you some help soon," I whispered, and his legs slid back down to the ground. Just then, Midnight's body visibly tensed. His right hind leg lifted off the ground and curled to his abdomen in what appeared to be a slow-motion version of an extreme muscle contraction.

"Nick, look!" Midnight's leg remained clenched to his abdomen long enough for us to wonder if it was a permanent alteration. "What's it doing?" I asked.

"I don't know," Nick said. As we gaped, the leg lowered gradually back down to the ground, and the tension that had seized Midnight's body released in a slow leak. Nick knelt and worked his hands over the length of the dog's body, talking softly as he felt for whatever he thought he might find. Midnight tensed again. My heart skipped.

"Something's really wrong," I said.

"Yeah," Nick said quietly, standing back as he watched Midnight's left hind leg lift in a contraction that mirrored the one we'd just witnessed. "I've never seen anything like this." Rather than waiting for the Monday appointment, he called the emergency number and took Midnight to the vet that day. It was nearly dark when he returned, and Midnight was not with him.

"What happened?" I asked. "What did they say?"

"Nothing," he said. "They took some blood and have to send it in to the lab for tests. They'll do X-rays next week."

"When will we know the results?"

"By mid-week," he said, looking out the kitchen window. "They're keeping him on watch until they know more." I wrapped my arms around Nick's torso and rested my chin on his slouched shoulder. We gazed out the window toward the kennel now missing one of its founding members.

A litany of exams, X-rays, and blood work uncovered nothing beyond a vitamin deficiency leading to Midnight's accelerated decline. "There's nothing they can do," Nick said after more than a week. His silence had grown disquieting. He moved Midnight from the kennel to our fenced-in yard for closer observation and comfort.

My work days in Park City blurred with thoughts of the waning dog in our backyard. I'd promised we would help him. I trusted that Nick would know what to do, but the news each night was the same. No answers had been found. We couldn't fix what we couldn't identify, and in the third week of his illness, Midnight stopped eating. Then he retreated to the darkened recesses under the porch, where his pitch-black coat fused with the shadows, and all we could see were the whites of his eyes on the rare occasions he inclined to open them.

Nick tried everything from T-bone steaks to female dogs to coax Midnight out from under that porch, but a stronger force called Midnight elsewhere. I came home from work one night, and he was gone. Just like that. He had died, Nick had buried him, and I never asked for details. I wasn't sure Nick would have the strength to provide them. I was sure I did not have the strength to listen.

At a young age, I'd intuited the emotional pitfalls of working with animals. When asked what I wanted to be when I grew up, "veterinarian" was my childhood response. I enunciated each syllable for enhanced dramatic effect—"vet-er-uh-nar-ee-an," I would respond to the popular question with pride. I was going to help animals. At some point I learned that veterinarians performed surgery on animals, which I suspected involved hurting them, and that sometimes, the animals died. This seemed counterproductive to my intentions. I recognized, prior to reaching double digits in age, that veterinary medicine would not be the perfect fit for a "sensitive" person like myself.

Over the years, intuition had dwindled to a less-trusted decision-making tool. So here I was now, living with a dog musher and his kennel full of sled dogs. While my childhood notions of working with animals had been theory based, Midnight's death showed firsthand what that life can entail. This is the life, I now understood, that I'd signed myself up for.

I dove back into my work after Midnight died, but by that time Sue was on her way out. Collective curiosity about the new marketing director electrified the office air. Though rumors buzzed, no one had concrete details to share. The owner had assumed control of the search, leaving Sue out of the process entirely, and for the first time, she could not supply me with helpful information. I would find out on my own soon enough.

"I think he's all icing and no cake!" A coworker said to me soon after my new boss had started. By that time I had other descriptive terms for him in mind. The marketing director and I shared a cubicle of approximately twelve by six feet, split down the middle by a small island. This had worked well for Sue and me, allowing us to share spontaneous ideas and discuss campaigns when inspiration struck. With my new boss, the setup acted more like a trap, locking me in a chamber of constant scrutiny and humiliation. My attempts to design flyers and advertisements were thwarted by his incessant chatter, which flip-flopped from self-aggrandizing to insulting the work I produced. I never knew which it was going to be from one day, or even one moment, to the next.

"That guy loved my ass!" he said to me during a lengthy narrative about a previous supervisor, in response to which I sat befuddled. *He must want me to like him*, I thought, my internal deliberation drowning out the rest of his story. *Why else would he brag so much?* But just when I thought he was warming up, he'd launch a dagger of criticism straight through the heart of my creative confidence.

The problem with his stories, in addition to disrupting my work time, was the fact that I felt rude if I did not look at him when he shared them. He'd launch into some random anecdote, and I'd continue working for as long as possible to imply that I did not have time to chat just then. Inevitably, he'd continue until I turned around to face him. It was his eyes that threw me off. Certain rodents, like possums or hamsters, can be cute, but if you stare at their beady eyes for too long, you're bound to walk away with an unsettled feeling. This was the sense I got from my boss. When I wasn't looking at him, I felt his black eyes boring into my back. I soon learned that his critical opinions were reaching the ears of the company owner whose confidence in me had been tenuous from the start.

"I'm concerned about the quality of your work," my new boss said one afternoon in reference to the first newspaper ad I'd allowed myself to feel pride in. Sue and I had conceptualized the Alpine Peak campaign in tandem. Based on our mutual ideas, I'd designed a full-page magazine ad, a full-page newspaper ad, and had written the slogan that prompted Sue to tell me slogans were a natural talent of mine. She'd asked her professional designer friends for feedback on my work, and they'd offered only minor suggestions. Alpine Peak was my gateway campaign. I'd gained the skills to build self-confidence on one of the company's most prestigious new accounts, and if the new marketing director didn't stop calling it Aspen Park, I felt certain Alpine Peak would not remain an account for much longer.

My hands were tied, and the new marketing director knew it. He rode, with audacious mastery, the golden chariot of unconditional trust, having been hand picked for the position by the owner of the company. His claims often contradicted what I'd learned from Sue, but my counter claims stood no chance of acceptance. The insults my new boss dispensed while hovering over my shoulder froze my productivity, and at least once a day, I'd escape to the basement and cry.

"You have to talk to the vice-president," one agent said after finding me sniffling in a darkened corner one morning, and I knew he was right. My glamorous Park City job had deteriorated to this decision point. I could walk away quietly or go over my new boss's head.

The day I sat across the table from the vice-president and exposed my feelings about the new marketing director, tears streamed down my cheeks. There was nothing she could do. Her loyalty, she said, lay with the president, and her support went to the marketing director he'd hired. She understood I could not remain in a position that pushed me to tears every day, and she offered to write a letter of reference before I left my glamorous Park City job forever, two weeks later.

When I told Nick what had happened, he held me in his arms as I sobbed. "The guy was an asshole," he said, his breath warm against my downturned head. "You don't deserve to be treated like that." I wanted to believe his assertions were true. "You'll find something better," he said. But this statement, I knew for a fact, was false.

Sadness can pass, I understood from experience. I wasn't as sure about depression, but the fact that I did not know how to differentiate between sadness and depression possibly worked in my favor. I thought

I might someday move beyond my exhaustion and stomach pain, now accompanied by feelings of worthlessness and soul-encompassing emptiness. My visits to the dogs still buoyed my spirits, which I took to mean hope existed. I could not yet grasp it, but I could intellectualize the probability of its presence in the world. I'd had hope once, so I might someday find it again, I thought as I sipped my glass of wine on the front porch swing of our trailer and gazed across Stringtown Road toward the kennel.

20

THE NEW JOB SEARCH routine involved waking up around 8:00 a.m., shuffling out to the kitchen to fix myself a cup of coffee, then retiring to my office where I'd alternate between examining the classifieds and rearranging my portfolio. I'd prepare a resume and cover letter on the rare occasion I happened upon a graphic design opportunity within reasonable range of my location and skill set.

Nick typically awoke before I did and hustled out to the living room to fix the fire in the woodburner before brewing the coffee. He'd then withdraw to his own office on the other side of the wall from mine. Throughout the morning, I'd occasionally hear an odd gurgling noise, like the sound of a fish tank filter, coming from Nick's office, and a curiously familiar odor would waft through the panel-thin wall. It must have been my life-long absence of pre-noon functional ability that caused a delay in my detective work. After more than a week, I finally connected the sounds and subsequent odor to past experience. My college boyfriend had, upon my first visit to his apartment, proudly presented a closet full of thriving marijuana plants. The bong, he'd explained, provided the purest pot-smoking experience. Nick must have felt the same, I now realized, because he started each day with this plant-based "Breakfast of Champions" via that very mechanism.

I'd always considered pot smoking to be an extracurricular activity, like drinking tequila shots, practiced only at parties or among intimate gatherings of friends. *Nobody smokes every morning*, I thought. Then again, if I hadn't witnessed the situation firsthand, I would not have believed the number of marathon cell phone conversations Nick engaged in daily. As I mulled over job listings, Nick talked on the phone. He'd pace up and down the hallway outside my office doorframe (the door itself having been a casualty of renovation during move-in week), rarely pausing between sentences for breath. I tuned out the details of his conversations, bearing little interest in the Internet plans he concocted with his virtual office mates as I contended with my own job-related concerns.

During those first few weeks of unemployment, the likelihood of incorporating a shower into my daily routine went from probable to possible. I adopted disturbingly similar practices to those Nick had honed to perfection over many years in a work-at-home setting. I'd sometimes hear him talking to himself through the wall between our offices. "I steeeeeenk!" he would say at a volume intended for sharing, and though it always sparked a giggle, I could not, in truth, disagree. I started calling him Stinky. Then he called me Stinky. We adopted the joint nickname so naturally that he once yelled "Hey Stink!" from the opposite end of a Smith's grocery store aisle in an attempt to draw my attention. The words drew more attention than he'd bargained for. As I turned my head to join the other shoppers in their search for the unfortunate person named "Stink," I found myself wondering, *What ever happened to "pretty girl"?*

One night in late winter, the sound of banshees screaming on the back porch jolted Nick and I out of a deep, 3:00 a.m. slumber. Katy and Chief whined and paced, pressing their noses into the crevice between the door and the floor with each distressing shriek.

"What the hell is that noise?" I whispered to Nick.

"I have no idea," he said, crawling out of bed and reaching for the door.

"Don't open it!" I said. "The dogs will go out."

Nick listened at the door for a while, but the source of the wails remained a mystery. The same banshees returned with their hair-bristling screams for several more nights.

After a week of this unholy night terror, I walked into the garage where Nick stood preparing food for the dogs. A pungent odor hung thick in the air.

"Oh my god," I said. "It's cats."

"What?"

"Cats," I repeated.

"What are you talking about?" Nick laughed.

"The banshees we've been hearing. They're cat fights. Can you smell that musky odor?"

"Yeah, it reeks in here. It's been getting worse and worse."

"It's cat spray."

"Yuck," he said.

"They must have moved into the garage when it got cold outside."

From that point forward, signs of the feline squatters grew more apparent. The tomcat showed himself first. Likely once a recognizable orange tabby, this cat appeared to have bargained for several lives in addition to the nine traditionally granted. His matted fur looked like well-traveled tumbleweed, and his left ear had been gnawed or otherwise torn partially off. Several critical teeth had gone missing, a circumstance made apparent when he stretched his mouth open to meow. Sometimes no sound emerged at all, which was almost more distressing than the times a rasping cough choked out, as if he were in need of a tracheotomy in addition to the lengthy list of reconstructive alterations he'd already undergone. Nick and I referred to this new beast as Orange Cat or Scabby Tabby, depending on our moods. The cat was an obvious rebel who lived in our garage on his own terms and timeline. When the weather warmed, he rambled on to the next adventure that called.

The other garage-invading feline proved more elusive. We caught occasional glimpses of this cat perched behind many layers of protective paraphernalia, including two forty-gallon dog food bins, a pile of plywood, and an old porcelain tub. Black as licorice and just as shiny, this cat emitted soft, melodious meows, which lured us toward the dark crevices of its hideout. Before we knew it, the meow would transform into a hiss threatening enough to prompt several steps backward. The alluring meow would return for a moment, only to be followed by another surprise warning.

Though we lacked faith in the black cat's mental stability, and the sight of Scabby Tabby inspired battling reactions of empathy and disgust, we feared the cats would starve in the frigid remains of winter. We purchased some cat food on our next trip to Smith's. This small act coaxed the black cat out of hiding, at which point we discovered it was also a male. Though the name Dr. Jekyll came first to mind, we thought it best not to name him at all. The last thing Nick and I needed, we both agreed, was the responsibility of another pet. As we took turns stroking the now affectionate cat's velvety coat, Nick referred to him as Little Cat, and the generic term stuck.

"Lee-tool caaat, lee-tool caaat," Nick would call as he poured the Friskies dry mix into a bowl, and our feline friend would emerge from hiding to rub his silky fur against Nick's ankles, softly purring with never a hiss to be heard again.

Being unemployed afforded more time to spend with the sled dogs, which I regarded as an unforeseen perk. Nick had moved the kennel from the original fenced-in area that was open to the elements into the semi-open portion of the barn that still had a roof and a wooden frame. To this new area, he'd added several truck loads of small stones amounting to a floor base conducive to cleanup by pitchfork, as opposed to garden shovel. He had also built or otherwise procured wooden houses for each of the dogs.

One afternoon, Nick returned from the kennel and burst through the front door to tell me he was taking Jax to the vet. Apparently, he'd misjudged the length of the dog chains in the new kennel. Rocky and Jax could just reach each other's snouts. As a result, Jax's snout had a gash down the left side straight through to his gums. He would need a lot of stitches.

A shy dog to begin with, Jax returned home in his protective plastic head cone still groggy from the anesthetic and bumping cone-first into everything. He was more than a little spooked when Nick put him in the backyard to recuperate. Because I feared the experience would shatter his trust in us and because my unemployed status provided me all the time in the world to do with as I pleased, I grabbed a book and a camp chair, and I set myself up as a daily fixture in the backyard with Jax.

For the first few days, he examined me from a distance, taking tentative steps toward me before losing his nerve and running off, to the best of his ability as a cone head. I sat in my camp chair, reading and pretending to ignore Jax's presence until curiosity overtook him, and he braved the unknown to investigate me up close. Each day he grew bolder, and by the end of the first week, he greeted me eagerly. Something in his eyes or in the casual way he now regarded me assured me that I'd earned Jax's trust. Why I needed it wasn't as clear. Perhaps the lack of ambivalence in dogs calls out to a person who is so lost she doesn't know she's lost. Watching over Jax prevented my ruminating on the negative aspects of my situation. This dog was also displaced, but it hadn't been his choice.

I studied Jax as he made his way around the yard, familiarizing himself with a new set of surroundings and growing accustomed to the human fixed in the same location in the middle of the yard each day. I watched this gray and white dog with his pale blue eyes, who was not only displaced, but also hurt, scared, and still trying his best to adapt. I'd never know how many unfamiliar situations Jax had been obliged to adapt to in his lifetime—how many families he'd lost and formed, then lost again.

Maybe this was my part to play, the part of nurturer in Nick's working dog world. I could attempt to balance Nick's utilitarian purposes with my unconditional love and support. As Nick pushed his dogs to be fast and strong, athletic and competitive, I would do my best to make sure they were happy. I would secretly watch over my fellow transients on weekend kennel visits, letting Nick know if anything seemed out of the ordinary. I was sure he'd be on top of most situations that arose, but on the off chance that he missed one, I'd be there. We were in Nick's dog mushing dream together, the sled dogs and I. This was the least and, at the same time, the best I could do.

I stroked Jax's chest as he raised his nose toward my face, exposing the blood-crusted tangle of stitches that adorned his swollen snout. As his face drew near to mine, the scent of carnage wafted up from his cone.

21

AFTER ALMOST TWO MONTHS of searching, I found a graphic design position at the local newspaper and publishing company just a few miles from our home. Gone were my salaried days of brainstorming campaigns for multimillion dollar properties, and in their place were time clock punching days of production work with limited original thought required. But I was desperate. I'd take what I could get and worry about advancement when I had the luxury of a steady income, even if that income was $10,000 a year less than I'd been making in Park City.

While I returned to full-time work, Nick better acquainted himself with our neighbors. The Gardenias, whose names we now knew were Dan and Kelli, ventured over for a visit one Saturday afternoon to request the use of their old garden in our new yard. Apparently the ground was still too hard from winter's chill for them to dig a fresh garden next door.

"Knock yourselves out," Nick told them, confident that we'd benefit from their hard work in the form of at least a few zucchinis. While we had them engaged in conversation, we asked our neighbors about the local nightlife. Our sporadic social activities had dwindled down to kennel visits and the occasional dinner out—just the two of us—since I'd left my Park City job. But Dan and Kelli confirmed that aside from Swiss Days and an annual rodeo, Heber City offered little in the form of entertainment.

"We were thinking about going to The Other End tonight if you want to come," Dan said.

"There's going to be a band." Kelli added.

"The other what?" Nick and I looked at each other.

"The bar," Dan said. "It's called The Other End."

We'd seen the bar Dan referred to and would have gladly ventured into the establishment ourselves if it hadn't been for the fact that bars in Utah required memberships, more like private clubs than the public bars

Nick and I were familiar with. On principle alone, Nick and I refused to spend hard-earned money on a membership just to get into a plain old bar. Our drink and tip money should suffice, we believed, as it did anywhere else we'd ever been. As a result of that belief, we spent our booze money at Smith's grocery store and our evenings drinking that booze in the isolation of our trailer. After eight months, the practice had grown tedious.

"We don't have a membership," Nick said.

"Why is it called The Other End?" I asked.

"You can go as our guests," Dan said, then he shrugged. "All I know about the name is there used to be another bar at the other end of town."

"Yeah, we'll definitely go," Nick said with a tad too much enthusiasm. "That sounds great!"

The Other End, Gardenias informed us as we perused the menu that evening, was known for its garlic burgers and fries. "You have to try their fry sauce," Dan said, and Nick and I both dropped our menus to gape.

Before I could get a word out, Nick leaned across the table toward Dan. "What is fry sauce?" he said. "And why is the entire state of Utah so obsessed with it?"

Almost everywhere Nick and I dined, the same question arose. "Do you want fry sauce with that?" the wait staff would ask, and our inquiry as to the ingredients prior to answering would elicit an obscure explanation that was impossible to decode. It was as if everyone in Utah's food industry had watched the same training video on how to describe fry sauce without divulging the ingredients, a practice that annoyed us both to distraction.

"It's just ketchup and mayonnaise," Kelli said.

"Why is it such a big secret?" Nick and I wanted to know, but our new friends could not speak to that question. Utah had its way of keeping outsiders out, Nick and I were learning, and the fry sauce secret served as one of many built-in mechanisms for doing so. Knowing the ingredients felt like a minor breakthrough. We'd breached a tiny part of Utah's covert culture wall, courtesy of our native neighbors. I ordered the garlic burger and fries with a double order of fry sauce, and after one taste, I slathered the fry sauce all over my burger and proceeded to devour the entire half-pound feast.

"I'm too full for beer," Kelli said, reading my mind as the band set up. "Let's do some tequila shots."

Several rounds later, the band wailed and the barroom rocked at full capacity. I wove through the crowds to the restroom, where the silence and fluorescent lights clashed with the blaring music and tequila still pulsing through my body. The contrast created a tenuous strip of altered reality, and I shook my head to clear the buzz before hovering over the seat in the stall, taking care to touch as few surfaces as possible. Two women entered the restroom, talking loudly about an ex-boyfriend or husband. I flushed and stepped out of the stall, at which point one of the women, still conversing with her friend in the other stall, hoisted her bare and, accordingly, grimy foot into the room's only sink. The foot on the bathroom floor was also bare, and no shoes appeared in the vicinity. I must have gawked as the woman picked something out of her toenail, but she did not acknowledge my presence with a glance or a pause in her amplified diatribe. I pulled myself together and made extreme haste out of there. The hand washing could wait for another time, and maybe even another sink.

I returned to the table flustered and blurted my twilight zone experience to the group. Nick scrunched his face in disgust, but the Gardenias remained unfazed. Dan shrugged, and Kelli's blank expression at the end of my rant indicated she was still waiting for the punch line. She turned to face the band with a barely perceptible eye-roll being the only indication she'd heard me.

I hope they don't think I'm a snob, I worried. Maybe all those tequila shots would make them forget I'd said anything. To be safe, I ordered another round.

The band improved as the alcohol flowed, and by the end of the third set, I found myself on the dance floor, my left arm looped around Dan's and my right arm around Kelli's, swaying to the music as if we were lifelong best friends. As the bar cleared out and the band packed their equipment, I crossed paths with the lead singer on the dance floor. I stopped to compliment her on the band's performance. Her rendition of "Magic Man" had rivaled Nancy Wilson's, and she seemed pleased to hear the comparison.

"Are you from around here?" I asked.

"New Jersey," she said. "We travel around a lot."

"I'm from back east too," I told her. "Pennsylvania."

"What brings you the whole way out here?" she asked.

"My boyfriend and I moved across the country so he could follow his dream of being a dog musher," I said, proudly alluding to my adventurous and, at the same time, supportive nature.

"Really?" She shifted her guitar from one hand to the other, then looked back at me. "What's your dream?" she asked.

"Well," I paused. "I'm a writer," I heard myself say, though I hadn't written much of anything since college. "But I can do that anywhere," I added, still supportive. Still adventurous.

"Hmph," she grunted, arcing her left eyebrow in a way I've always wished I could. "Good luck," she said brushing past me on her way to the door.

"Thank you," I said, but that "Magic Man" singer was out of earshot, and my words hung abandoned in the air before the glaring lights and echoing last sounds of the closing bar swallowed them whole.

In addition to bare feet in the bar bathroom, more than a few elements of Utah's lifestyle etiquette hovered beyond my comfort zone. I didn't think I'd ever get used to bare feet walking down the aisles of Smith's grocery store, nor could I fathom or otherwise condone the shirtless male torsos which frequented any number of indoor public establishments. I had to surmise that these people had never heard of the "No shirt, No shoes, No service" stipulations that ruled in the east. And if I heard the words "Oh my heck," one more time, I was liable to let loose with a slew of profanity that would make George Carlin blush from beyond. "Oh my heck." What the hell was that supposed to mean? People said it all the time. *Why don't you say holy shit, or I'll be damned, like a normal person?* I wanted to say, *for chrissake.*

I was careful, after the Gardenias' reaction at the bar, to keep my opinions to myself or to share them exclusively with Nick, who I knew felt the same way I did. We became exclusive confidantes in the fine art of Utah bashing. I'd never forget the first time Rose insisted we water our grass.

"She asked us to what?" I said, not believing my ears.

"We have to water the grass," Nick replied.

"But it hasn't rained in months. Aren't we in a drought?" Back east it seemed like they declared a drought emergency if it didn't rain for two weeks. "We can't waste water just to make our grass green," I counter-insisted.

"I know," Nick agreed. "I don't know what the fuck these people are thinking," he said, as he went outside to water the grass in the middle of another flesh-searing, bone-dry Utah day.

22

MY BROTHER AND HIS GIRLFRIEND embarked on a cross-country road trip from their home in Wilmington, Delaware that August. Their plan was to visit as many national parks as they could squeeze into a three-week time period while exploring the many other wonders of the American West. Our little trailer in Midway, Utah sat close enough to the path between the Rocky Mountain and Grand Canyon National Parks to land on their destination list. Plus, we were family. They couldn't, in good faith, pass within a hundred mile radius of our new location without stopping for a visit.

Brian and I had shared over the years what might be interpreted as a complicated sibling relationship. This basically allowed for unlimited harassment on his part but came with an unspoken pact of his protection against similar treatment by others. The older we grew, the less he tormented me, and somewhere around puberty, he stopped picking on me altogether. We would frequently cross paths at those weekend keg parties throughout high school. He'd nod across the room in acknowledgment of my presence, then we'd proceed with our respective games of quarters or thumper or asshole or whatever else we'd invented to inspire us to chug beer faster on any such occasion. Part of me felt safer drinking beer out on Eagleton mountain in the summertime or in a variety of random strangers' homes in winter, knowing my big brother was there too.

After high school, we saw each other less frequently but engaged in actual conversations when we did. We'd catch up on holidays over turkey and Chianti or chicken divan and chardonnay. By traditional American standards, we may not have had what most would consider to be a close relationship, but to us, sibling status seemed as good a reason as any for a visit.

By the time they reached our Midway trailer, four days after leaving Delaware, Brian and Sarah had traveled almost 3,000 miles and had already visited several national parks. Nick and I relieved them of their sightseeing frenzy with a quiet day at the Midway trailer-stead and dog-kennel. We prepared lunch—our new favorite meal of lime-grilled chicken with mango and black bean salsa accompanied by garlic mashed potatoes. Then Nick and I ransacked our closets for kennel attire so that Brian and Sarah could meet all the dogs. It didn't occur to us that they may not be interested in meeting all the dogs until we reached the kennel and Sarah politely opted to remain outside the fence.

Later that day, we walked around the property in the bright, Utah sunshine, stopping at the garden to tell Brian and Sarah about the massive zucchini our neighbors had grown and given us the year before. Brian talked about his recipe for fried zucchini, which reminded me of a dinner our grandma and grandpa had sometimes prepared when we were growing up. Breaded steak and potatoes was a meal reserved for special occasions, but when those occasions came around, the whole family was called into action. Grandma would crush the saltine crackers between two sheets of wax paper with a rolling pin then pour the crumbs into a bowl. Dad would dip sliced potatoes in egg wash before Brian and I took turns pressing them into the breadcrumbs. The breaded potatoes went onto a plate, which, when filled with one layer, would be passed to Grandpa at the stove. With a fork, he'd place each slice into the frying pan, sizzling with oil, and turn them regularly as they browned. Cooked potatoes were piled in pyramid formation and placed in the warm oven. After all the potatoes had been fried, the same routine would repeat with the steak. Then Brian and I would mix the leftover egg and cracker crumbs into a gluey mass, which we'd flatten into patties for Grandpa to fry in the darkened oil. The egg patties, by way of there being so few, were our favorite part of the meal.

"We should make fried zucchini for dinner," I suggested, my mouth watering from the steak and potato memory. Brian agreed, and we all hopped into the Jeep to purchase ingredients. We took a few detours on our way to and from the grocery store to show Brian and Sarah a few places of interest such as where I worked, The Other End, and my personal favorite based on name alone, Dairy Keen.

That night Brian and I breaded and fried a pyramid of zucchini slices, following the exact method we'd witnessed and practiced over so many years at Grandma and Grandpa's house. We scraped together enough egg patties for Nick and Sarah to try, and the rest of the meal included leftovers of lime-grilled chicken and salsa, to which we'd added the option of flour tortillas during our grocery store run. We ate and drank and laughed as we shared our respective travel stories.

"We drove for twenty-four hours!" Sarah admitted after several bottles of beer.

"What?" I said.

"Your brother wouldn't stop." Her eyes assumed flying saucer dimensions.

"Why the hell not?" Nick laughed.

"There's nothing to see in the middle of the country," Brian stated, and Sarah's saucer shaped eyes rolled toward me.

"Hey, we stopped," I shrugged in response. "But then again, we weren't really on a timetable." Now I rolled my eyes and rose to clear the table as Sarah giggled at our respective predicaments.

"Well, you can rest here," Nick said to our guests, and I agreed that they'd better. My brother was more bull-headed than I remembered, and I had to wonder what else was in store for his girlfriend as they continued their race around the western part of the country.

After Nick washed the dishes, leaving the frying pan in the sink to soak, he pulled out the futon bed in the living room for Brian and Sarah to sleep on. We had plans to surprise them with an extravagant brunch the next day, but we were all too full to think about food just then. We'd save that topic for morning, Nick and I agreed after saying goodnight to our guests.

I awoke the next morning to my brother scrubbing the frying pan with pit bull determination.

"What are you doing?" I asked, staring at the sparkling pan.

"We made grease stains in your Calphalon pan. I'm trying to get them out," he said, still scrubbing.

"Those stains have been there since the first time Nick and I made rosemary and garlic pork chops," I said. "Thanks, though. That's the cleanest I've seen that pan since we bought it." Brian placed the pan on the counter as I turned from the sink. "We're taking you to brunch," I said over my shoulder as I made my way toward the bathroom for a shower.

Sue had told me about the Sundance Sunday brunch while I worked at the real estate company, and Nick and I had partaken twice since that time. The brunch was extravagant not only for the cost in relation to our annual incomes, but also for the astounding display of culinary perfection that graced the rustic Sundance dining room. I knew my brother would appreciate the gourmet buffet at least as much as I did, and the ride over the Wasatch mountain range from Heber City through the expansive aspen forests into Sundance, provided a feast of its own for the eyes.

As the high-noon sun beamed its rays in stoic columns down to the forest floor, the white aspen trunks reached up, stretching in the opposite direction toward the sky. Trees and light embraced at the canopy level, and those of us on the ground were treated to a blanket of golden warmth. The silence of the half-hour ride indicated to me that Brian and Sarah shared our appreciation for this glorious mountain trail through paradise.

At brunch, we feasted on eggs Benedict dripping with buttery hollandaise, salmon poached to such a peak of perfection that it melted at the touch of the tongue, and succulent roast beef still steaming when carved upon request. Toward the end of the meal, I glanced at Sarah's plate and saw the product of a dream-come-true.

"What's that?" I asked, pointing.

"I think its stuffed French toast," she said. I continued to stare at her plate. "It's right over there in the corner." She pointed to a food warmer on the other side of the room.

"I didn't know they stuffed French toast." I said. "What do they stuff it with?" I asked, my eyes still glued to her plate.

"It's some kind of cream cheese mixture," she began, but I was already out of my chair with my plate in hand and headed for the food warmer on the other side of the room.

Any attempts at normal functioning after the Sundance Sunday brunch were in vain, Nick and I knew, so we suggested taking a ride on the chair lift to see the view from the top of the mountain. About halfway up, as we dangled from our seats a few hundred feet from the earth, a tidal wave of nausea arose in my gut and surged into my chest. The mountain range surrounded us like a row of teeth, and the valley loomed below like an open gullet.

"This is gorgeous!" Sarah yelled from the chair in front of us just as my vision blurred.

"Oh my god," I moaned, grabbing my stomach.

"Are you O.K.?" Nick asked, simultaneously giving Sarah the thumbs up as he flashed a wide grin and nodded in her direction.

"No," I said. "I ate way too much." I leaned forward to shift my weight, and the nausea rose to my throat. "Why did I have to eat that French toast?" I said more to myself than to Nick. "I was already full."

"I know," Nick said. "We always overdo it when we come here."

"I've never felt like this," I said, pulling on the waistband of my shorts. There seemed to be a balloon in my stomach that was inflating by the second.

"Is there anything I can do?" Nick asked. I took a slow, deep breath in an effort to control my heart palpitations.

"I don't think so," I said. Nick patted my leg, and I groaned in response.

The ride home over bumpy mountains and windy roads caused me to break out in a sweat. Brian made fun of me for eating so much, but intestinal distress prevented my usual ability to muster the self-deprecating variety of humor to which my own family had conditioned me.

It might be funny later, I thought, *if I can keep my heart from exploding right now.* The contents of my stomach felt like molten lava. As Brian produced another wise-crack, I wondered how funny he'd find it if that molten lava were to erupt in the car. Had I opened my mouth to ask, I feared that it might.

The violence of my reaction on this occasion threw me off. I'd overeaten plenty of times in my life—enough to consider it a nearly perfected skill—and I'd never felt anything like the heart palpitations, shooting pain, nausea, bloating, and sweating of this reaction.

It was the last time I'd ever partake of the Sundance Sunday brunch. A few months later, Nick's friend would come to help him build a support system under the section of the trailer that was sinking beneath the river rock corner where the woodburner stood. Nick treated his friend to the Sundance feast that weekend, but I was under the weather with stomachaches that had grown progressively more debilitating and was not well enough to join them.

That afternoon with Brian and Sara, we made it back to Midway without incident, but my stomach convulsions continued into the evening.

The next day, I opted out of breakfast and tiptoed around the futon on my way out the door to work as Brian and Sarah slept. Midway through morning, a heaviness settled in my chest, and around 2:00 in the afternoon, I realized they were gone. My brother had left me in Utah, and I had no idea when I'd see my family again.

I returned from work to an empty trailer. I pulled a pair of Carhartts over my clothes and walked out the door to the kennel where Nick was making his cleaning rounds. The dogs greeted me as they always did, with boundless joy and happiness. They didn't know I was depressed. They didn't know what depressed was. *This is my family now,* I thought, hoping to catch their exuberance like I might catch the flu. I stroked Jax's head and braced myself for the other dogs, who launched themselves at my body in playful greeting. As Nick walked around with his pitchfork, loading the waste into buckets, I watched all the dogs interact. Each had been uprooted from its original home and many from more homes than that. They wouldn't recognize their siblings if they ran into them on the dog sled trail, I realized. Still, they seemed happy. *These sled dogs have the key,* I thought, *the key to happiness.* And I wondered if they might, someday, share it with me.

23

"HAVE YOU SEEN LITTLE CAT?" Nick said as he came in from the garage one day.

"No." I looked up from my computer. "But I haven't been out back all week. Can't you find him?"

"I haven't seen him in about three days."

"He's a stray cat," I said. "Don't you think he's probably off hunting?"

"He's usually around in the afternoon." Nick stood quietly for a moment. Then he turned and walked back to the garage.

I was working in my office two weeks later when Nick cracked open the door and yelled, "Little Cat is back!" I rushed outside.

"He's up there," Nick pointed to a shadow in the garage rafters where a pair of green eyes peered down at us. "He won't come out."

"What's that smell?" I said.

"What smell?"

"It smells like," I paused. "Lighter fluid?" I looked at Nick. "Some kind of fuel. Can you smell it?"

"Yeah," Nick said. "I didn't notice it until now."

"Have you been using something like that in here? Gasoline or anything?"

"No, I was just getting the dog food ready."

I told Nick I'd stay in the garage to keep Little Cat company while he went across the street to feed the dogs. Then I sat on the steps leading from the deck into the garage.

"What's the matter Little Cat?" I cooed. "Come and see me." I talked for several minutes in my most soothing voice with Little Cat staring silently down at me. He finally emerged from the shadows to pace along the rafters.

He must be hungry, I thought. I filled Little Cat's bowl and sat back down on the steps, holding the bowl up and shaking it for Little Cat to hear. He stopped in his tracks, stared at the food for a moment, then made his way down from the rafter. I placed the bowl on the step beside me. As he crouched to eat, a noxious odor rose from his fur, and I saw that an oily substance coated his back.

"Oh my god, Little Cat," I whispered, "What happened to you?" He crunched greedily, purring as he ate, and I leaned in for a better look. A wispy combination of damaged follicles and budding new growth replaced his once full coat. Pockets of buttery puss punctuated the exposed inflamed flesh and oozed between thick cakes of scabs. The horror show extended from the base of his tail to the tips of his shoulder blades. "Poor Little Cat," I whispered, willing myself not to pet him. At the sound of my voice, he purred louder.

When Nick entered the garage after feeding the dogs, Little Cat raced back up to the rafters.

"Something bad happened," I said. He looked at me. "Little Cat has lighter fluid all over his back, and it looks like he was burned."

"Oh my god," Nick said. "Are you sure?"

"Stay here for a minute. He'll come back down if you sit still."

Nick sat beside me, and this time Little Cat emerged from hiding more quickly. Nick took one look, said, "I'm calling the cops," then marched inside, slamming the door behind him.

"Someone tortured my cat," I heard him say through the paper-thin wall, knowing he was pacing the hall as he spoke. "I want to file a report, and I want someone to come over here and investigate." After talking with the police for about five minutes, Nick called the vet's emergency line. The police officer arrived while he was out picking up the prescribed antibiotic.

To ensure that the officer would see Little Cat's burns, we'd confined him in Katy's plastic dog crate and placed it outside on the front porch. I sat on the artificial grass carpeting next to Little Cat, who paced within his thirty-six-inch prison. The sound coming from the kennel was closer to a growl than a purr. I remained in my seated position, hugging my knees to my chest as I explained the situation to the officer in a distant voice I hardly recognized as my own. I did not wipe the tears from my cheeks as I spoke, and I lifted my head only once to witness the officer bobbing his head in response to my story. He shifted his feet, and I lowered my head back down to my knees. The Jeep pulled into the driveway. Nick stormed onto the porch and repeated the story in a much different tone.

"What kind of a sick person would do something like this?" he said to the officer, who shook his head and muttered a variation of the same sentence he'd been feeding to me.

"We'll get the report on file," he said, and Nick continued his rant.

"Do you see cases like this a lot?" Nick questioned rhetorically. "I can't even believe anyone would do something this horrible."

The officer looked at the ground and, again, shook his head. "We'll file that report for you," he said. After fifteen minutes, Nick had exhausted attempts to elicit anything other than the canned response. He let the officer off the hook by handing over the fully completed report.

The officer speed-walked to his car. "O.K. then, we'll get this filed," he said, holding up the paperwork as he crouched through the driver-side door. He'd scarcely glanced at Little Cat during the full half-hour visit.

We told the Gardenias about Little Cat's experience later that week.

"People do stuff like that all the time," Dan said. Even Kelli seemed unfazed.

"Sometimes people shoot cats around here," she said.

"Why would they do that?" Nick's voice elevated.

Dan shrugged and walked across the living room to change the CD. "They just do."

"Well, that's bullshit," I said, grinding the conversation to a halt. The sadness that had engulfed me since the day we'd found Little Cat finally festered into righteous anger. Nick placed his hand on my thigh in solidarity, though his anger had long since burned itself down.

Kelli changed the subject by asking Nick and I about our hometowns. She said she was from southern Utah, and Dan hailed from exactly where we were sitting. Nick and I told them about the section of the Appalachian chain that rolled through our home base in central Pennsylvania. But after feasting our eyes on the behemoths comprising the Wasatch portion of the Rockies, we hesitated to use the term "mountains" in description. Our native land featured its share of pastorally pretty elements, but the most effective reference point was always its status as the home of Penn State football. After seeing the flicker of recognition in Dan's eyes, we told them about a lesser known institution with regard to the area—a Fourth of July fireworks display that consistently ranked among the top ten in the country. This time, Kelli's eyes flickered.

"Wow," she said and looked at Dan. "If their Fourth of July is that big, I wonder what their *twenty*-fourth is like." Nick and I looked at each other.

"They probably don't know about that," Dan said.

"What are you talking about?" Nick asked.

"It's a Utah thing," Dan said. "Pioneer Day. It's when the Mormons entered the state."

"And that's a bigger celebration than the Fourth of July?" I said.

"Yeah, we hardly see any fireworks on the Fourth," Kelli said.

"Wow." Nick looked at Dan. "That is unbelievable."

Dan smiled. "That's Utah."

The fact that my Utah friends were the first to point out the idiosyncrasies of their native state struck me as potentially significant. One of my coworkers frequently chuckled as we worked, "We should get T-shirts made that say, 'Welcome to Planet Utah.'" Every time she said it, I wholeheartedly agreed.

The twenty-fourth of July conversation really threw me for a loop. *How could anyone think the state they live in is more important than the country?* I wondered, but it wasn't a question I was willing to ask that night at Dan and Kelli's with the tension of the cat-torturing discussion still lingering in the air.

24

UTAH EXHIBITED ALL THE QUALITIES of a mirage. Golf course green lawns defied the laws of the desert in gorgeous aberration, while the acute edges, contrasting angles, and fiery hues of the landscape converged in a breathtaking oasis that veiled an underlying danger. Rather than existing in harmony with nature, living in Utah felt like fighting against the odds for survival. I'd seen where people built houses—right in the middle of the native brush. The kind that needs to burn to regenerate as part of its natural life cycle. Multimillion dollar homes sat in brush kindling just waiting to catch a spark from the sun and combust into raging, seed-flinging flames. I sometimes dreamed of those flames coming after me, reaching down a nonexistent hill toward our trailer. Each time I dreamed it, the flames inched closer.

In summer, the steadfast sun could sear to a crisp anything that sat too long in its path. And the "good powder" winters people flocked to enjoy might just as easily swallow them up. Nick and I frequently awoke on winter mornings to explosions far off in the distance. These "triggers," we learned, were timed to incite avalanches which were bound to occur on their own but which, on their own, had no sense of the skiers and snowboarders they might bury. I heard on the news that a couple from New England had failed to collect their toddler from the day care center of a ski resort. They had dropped the child off before hitting the slopes and, according to eyewitness reports, ventured into an off-limits area of the mountain. Search parties had dispatched, but I never learned whether or not the child's parents were found.

Utah's beauty ranked in the terrifying category to be respected in the same way a God-fearing Catholic respects his Maker. Losing sight of the nature of your relationship with either force might land you in an avalanche or careening off an icy mountain roadway. Beyond treacherous landscape and weather conditions, the multitude of stories I'd heard of people with cancer caught up with my conscious awareness about a year after moving to Utah. Sue had talked of her sister's battle with cancer, which resulted in multiple surgeries that had permanently altered her face. Before Sue left the company, she learned that her brother had cancer as well. In fact, most of the people I'd met in Utah had at least one close relative who had previously battled or was currently battling cancer. If the same were true back east, I'd somehow avoided awareness, and I wondered if this Utah cancer situation was as bleakly unusual as it seemed.

I saw more people with prosthetic limbs during my first year in Utah than I'd seen in my entire previous life. Everything from sophisticated prosthetics that looked bionic and maybe *did* cost six million dollars, to the wooden stump variety that replaced Kelli's leg from just below the knee joint, cohabitated with their biological counterparts throughout Park City and surrounding areas. Neither Nick nor I had wanted to pry for information about Kelli's leg, but one day, after joining them for a hearty meal of Dan's famous meatloaf burgers, the conversation took a turn toward the hazards of driving to and from Park City in winter.

"It was black ice," Kelli said. "We were going up Park City Mountain and slid out of control."

"We both landed outside the Jeep." Dan joined in. "One of the hubcaps flew off the tire and rolled through Kelli's leg. Sliced it right off."

"Dan died," Kelli said. Nick and I looked at Dan to make sure we were still talking about the same Dan.

"What?" we said in unison.

"He died," she repeated. "They did CPR and tried to bring him back, and when I saw them put that sheet over his head, I started screaming. He could take my leg but he wasn't taking Dan from me." *Was she talking about God?*

"What happened?" Nick asked.

"He came back to life," Kelli said, taking a hit from the bowl she'd been packing and passing it over to Nick.

"I just started breathing again," Dan said.

Nick and I sat in silent shock. They'd been driving a Jeep Wrangler, much like the one Nick drove now, when the accident occurred.

We later learned that Dan had hovered dangerously close to death's doorway on several other occasions during his job as a stonemason. One time, he told us, he'd been standing on scaffolding with his brother and a hefty supply of super-sized boulders when the scaffolding tipped over. Dan and his brother hit the ground first and lay frozen while giant boulders rolled off the scaffolding and crashed all around them. By the time we met him, Dan was counting his lives. According to Kelli, he was up to number eight.

The Gardenias taught us about the two kinds of people at the opposite ends of the Utah spectrum—the Mormons and the Jack-Mormons—all of whom had been born into the Mormon religion, some of whom had chosen to stray from the church. Dan and Kelli were of the Jack variety, which they explained was the farthest away from the accepted Mormon lifestyle. I knew Dan and Kelli threw some wild parties (full details of which I was not privy), but it wasn't until Kelli revealed that Nick and I were the most "normal" of all their friends that I realized I may not be working with the full picture. I'd always wanted to be normal and had striven hard all my life to do so. But I couldn't, under any imagined circumstances, place the word normal in the same room with Nick. Maybe not even in the same city.

Regardless of our normalcy, the Gardenias took us under their native Utah wing. They invited us over for dinner, to parties, and out to the bar, making sure we weren't unanimously shunned during our time there. I did find a few girlfriends at work who hovered closer to the middle of the Mormon versus Jack-Mormon spectrum. Both Lena and Jennifer—also graphic designers—had jumped off the Mormon train before it arrived at its final, one-way destination. Still, the passenger cars were intimately familiar to them.

Something about native Utahans struck me as impossible to define. They seemed to share a common secret that an outsider like me stood no chance of accessing. It didn't matter how much time I spent with my new friends. An unspoken divide stood between us. Perhaps the divide stemmed from the fact that, as the Gardenias had informed us, most people in Utah were born into the Mormon faith. Though I lacked concrete details on its history and doctrines, the functional value of the religion did present itself to me one afternoon at work.

The company owners had recently recruited the daughter of a family friend, an occurrence I was starting to recognize as a hiring pattern. The company was family owned, and management-level positions were held by family members. They kept a couple of people on staff who knew the layout tools and intricacies of prepress work but seemed to hire unskilled laborers, often in the form of friends' children, to help out with production work like updating basic forms and business cards. A few lunchtime conversations with my coworkers confirmed that there were no advancement opportunities with this company. As a result, I was already browsing the classifieds for other options.

The girl they'd most recently hired was twenty-two years old and kept, for the most part, to herself. Lena and I were discussing the Little Cat situation, questioning how anyone could perform such horrific acts on a fellow living creature, when I glanced across the room to find our young coworker staring at us.

"How do you guys do it?" she said. Lena and I shifted our attention, waiting for the rest of the question.

"How do we do what?" Lena chuckled. Her laugh always conjured an image in my mind of a cherub with an impish twinkle in its eye, pointing an arrow at someone else's rear end.

"You both seem to have such strong values and good ethics," our coworker said. Lena and I glanced at each other, then back at her. "How do you know what to believe," she earnestly continued, "without the church to tell you?"

I sat perfectly still, mouth slightly ajar, absolutely silent. Lena burst out laughing.

25

IN FALL OF 2000, with help from his father, Nick traded his Jeep for a swank new truck—a Chevy 2500 Dually with an extended cab. Stretched in silver decal along each side of the metallic midnight truck, a team of sprinting dogs pulled a sled, behind which the words "SnowDog Racing & Touring" appeared with all relevant contact information. We said goodbye to the Wrangler, and I noted the degree of ease with which the wooden dog box graced the bed of this luxurious Chevy.

Around the same time, Nick acquired two more dogs, Buster and Sandy. Buster's coat was the color of buttered popcorn and felt like plush down feathers. He was lean and graceful with dark button eyes that resembled those of a teddy bear. The other newcomer was long in the torso and sturdier than Buster. Sandy's short, coarse coat was closer to white, and her wide face featured soft brown eyes topped by one erect ear and another that tipped over the side of her head.

Sandy warmed up to me after a few weekend visits, but Buster proved more reserved. He would venture toward me while I played with the other dogs, sometimes sneaking within inches behind me. The moment I acknowledged his presence, he'd bolt in the other direction then complete a wide circle and repeat the performance. I felt his feathery coat on a few occasions, petting him lightly as he stood still as a statue, muscles taut and ready to sprint, which he did after a few seconds each time. Buster acquiesced to Nick's advances, whom he must have accepted as the alpha male, and the SnowDog team made fast work of inducting Buster and Sandy into the hierarchy of the established pack.

While Nick maintained his utilitarian outlook with regard to the sled dogs, I adhered to my secret role, loving them sans interest in their athletic abilities or expectations of their mushing performances. Not only was the pretense of my belonging in Nick's dog mushing world steadily deteriorating, but everything from my career to my health seemed to be backtracking beyond my control. Performing the role of nurturer distracted my mind from these potentially distressing facts, even if that role was self-appointed.

Nick took good care of his dogs, feeding them special diets at different times of the year based on variables like weather and training regimens; exercising them and cleaning the kennel twice a day; making sure their water bowls stayed full; taking them to the vet when they were sick; and keeping up with all necessary vaccinations. I knew he was spending more than every penny he had on those dogs, a fact that warmed my heart.

For all his efforts, Nick had yet to provide a dog sled tour to a paying customer. He still hadn't met all the regulations or acquired the proper permits to run his business. In anticipation of his eventual success, I designed business cards and rack cards for SnowDog Racing & Touring, and I wrote an article about the company for the winter issue of the magazine published by my employer.

"You can write for me any time!" the company owner said with a smile after reading the copy. He'd never shown such fervor for my design work. It came as a relief, though, to know I could whip out my writing skills, as planned, and still produce something of quality. I thought back to that night at the bar when the singer had asked, "What's your dream?" The question had vexed me since, and I wasn't sure why. Surely, this article substantiated the "I'm a writer, but I can do that anywhere" response. Still, my smugness felt fragile, like a hollowed-out shell.

"All you ever wanted to do was write stories," my mother had said to me, long after I'd given up the practice. But that was a different kind of writing. A junior high English teacher once rolled her eyes at my enthusiasm to read one of those stories, and I'd never raised my hand to share again. My self-consciousness sprouted that day and bloomed until no room remained for anything else. My stories, I realized in hindsight of my teacher's response, were useless and unwanted products of the overblown confidence of a self-absorbed child. The last entry I'd written in my still hidden journal sprawled in all caps across a two-page spread: I AM AFRAID TO WRITE.

But I wasn't afraid anymore. I had written plenty of articles since then, including this recent magazine feature. At least I was writing something, I rationalized to the long-gone singer, whose name I would never know.

Nick and I had set ourselves up with matching dishware, a respectable set of cutlery, and Calphalon cookware courtesy of the Park City Outlets and other surrounding area stores. We'd traveled to Salt Lake City for living room and bedroom furniture, gravitating toward the same sofa in a warehouse filled with hundreds of others and agreeing on the queen-sized Simmons Beauty Rest the moment our backs hit the showroom mattress. This compatibility in decorative taste backfired when we both chose the same bedroom dresser, but a brief conversation concluded in agreement that practicality trumped decorum when it came to such matters. We each felt we needed the drawer space afforded by the largest dresser in the warehouse, and two identical dressers in the same room was certainly classier than one large dresser, one small dresser, and a permanent pile of homeless clothes. Besides, we reasoned prior to solidifying the purchase, no one would be judging our bedroom furniture located at the back end of the cardboard shoe box we called home.

Weekly jaunts to the grocery store saw us strolling up one aisle and down the next, grabbing whatever tasty looking treats caught our eyes as we passed. Trips to the Park City liquor store were handled in the same fashion, albeit on a monthly basis. We'd typically finish shopping at either store when the cart was full, and two hundred or so dollars later, we'd venture home with most of the food we thought we needed to survive for the upcoming week or with the variety of beverages that would carry us through to the following month.

On most nights I'd cook a simple dinner after coming home from work. Sometimes Nick would make garlic and rosemary chicken, which he taught me to prepare as well. I learned to choose the components of our meals by varying the color palettes. "The more colorful your food is, the more nutrition it has," Nick said his mother always said, reinforcing my perception of the maternal origin of his wisdom.

After dinner, Nick would place our plates on the floor for Katy and Chief to lick clean before we loaded them into the dishwasher. This practice had not originated with his mother, and it never failed to turn my stomach. On the occasions I retrieved the dishes from the floor, the tactile sensation redirected my brainwaves from wherever they'd been enjoying themselves to the renewed shock at how thoroughly canine saliva coated the surface on which we repeatedly placed our dinner. Each time, I wondered how something that looked so clean could feel so slimy, like moss on a river rock. Nick refused to part with this habit, which he said replaced the effort and water it would take to rinse the dishes by hand. I acquiesced, adding this practice to a growing list of those I endeavored to live with by willfully suppressing the thoughts of them.

If I were to rank by discomfort level, saliva-coated plates fell lower on the list than the gun under the mattress. The location of the gun had also been my compromise after discovering, to my horror, that Nick had been sleeping with it under his pillow. I'd walked into the bedroom one afternoon and found him cleaning the largest revolver I'd ever seen. It looked like it belonged in Wyatt Earp's wild west or some turn-of-the-century military museum.

"What the hell is that?" I screeched.

"It's a Colt .45," he said as if it were common knowledge.

"O.K.," I took a deep breath. "What exactly is it doing in our bedroom?"

"I keep it under the pillow in case someone breaks in at night."

"We have two loud dogs who will, no doubt, wake us if there's an intruder."

"That's when the bastard can talk to the end of this barrel," Nick said, pointing the massive revolver at the wall with affected bravado.

"That thing goes under the bed. I am not getting my head blown off in the middle of the night."

"I keep the safety on..."

"Under the bed. And if anyone ever brings kids over to visit, that gun will have to be locked up." As a consenting partner in this relationship, I might be required to accept some unanticipated lifestyle elements, I thought as I stormed out of the bedroom, but no child was getting shot on my watch. That's where I drew the line.

Nick typically fell asleep on the couch around 7:00 o'clock, whether we'd eaten at home or at the Gardenias'—two equally frequent events. Katy and Chief would curl up on the floor by our feet at either location. If home, we'd be watching one of the seven channels we received through the antennae the Gardenias had installed when they lived in the trailer, usually whatever sitcom had claimed the prime eastern time slot, when Nick would invariably start to snore. I'd make a few efforts to wake him while I watched TV. Around 10:00 or 11:00 o'clock, I'd nudge him and say I was going to bed. Shortly thereafter, Nick would shuffle back to the bedroom, slide under the covers, and shimmy his way backward to my side of the bed. He'd snuggle against me, tucking into the fetal position so my body enfolded his like a cocoon.

One afternoon, the Gardenias invited us to a party at their friends' home just outside of town. It would beat another Saturday night of sipping pseudo-beer in the trailer, we agreed and accepted the invitation. Though we hadn't yet met the hosts of this party, they welcomed Nick and me just as all of the Gardenias' friends had. We recognized a few people we'd previously met, and we passed the afternoon chatting with them and tossing a tennis ball for the hosts' little terrier to chase in the backyard.

As the party wound down and guests filtered out, we stayed among the late-night stragglers, converging on the back porch for one more nightcap. The conversation turned to the topic of children—the ones people had and the ones they hoped to have in the future. Thinking I could avoid commenting on the subject, I quietly sipped my beer and periodically nodded or smiled or furrowed my brow to display interest in the offspring-inspired anecdotes. Positive my pretend-listening skills would deter anyone from distracting me with a side conversation, I'd almost convinced myself that the woman speaking into my left ear had not been actively trying to redirect my attention for the past five minutes. As one guest's story ended, so did my cover. The woman, whom I'd somehow failed to meet during the course of the day, now nudged my shoulder.

"Do you have any kids?" she asked.

"Me? Oh no. Nope. I don't have any," I answered barely glancing at her and hoping another conversation would ignite somewhere else in the circle.

"When are you gonna have some?" she continued, at which point I resigned to having been hooked through the nostril and reeled unwillingly into this ill-fated discussion. I leaned back and turned to fully face her for the first time.

"I don't plan to have any kids," I said.

"What?" The stranger's face reflected the satanic horns that had apparently sprouted through my forehead.

"I've never had that maternal instinct..."

"Well, you just haven't met the right man yet," she comforted before I could finish my thought. I looked at Nick, who was sitting immediately to my right. He showed no signs of having heard.

The conversation clung to me long after the party. When I least expected it, the woman's declaration would float to the surface of my mind, followed by the familiar face-burning flush that passive-aggressive accusations or otherwise personal insults tended to provoke, especially after I'd failed to retaliate with a clever response. *Who the hell did she think she was?* I thought every time the memory struck. *Not everyone wants kids. Not everyone has to have kids!*

I had no idea why the comment still irked me, but the fact that it did really irked me. This train of thought led me to question another phenomenon that currently plagued me. Every once in a while I'd hear a song on the radio that reduced me to tears for no reason whatsoever. I'd be driving on my way to or from work when this blubbering weakness would most often strike. The songs eliciting this reaction were sappy love songs that I didn't even like. Whitney Houston's version of "I Will

Always Love You" was the worst offender. I hated that song. And every time I heard it, I bawled my eyes out.

Lately, I found myself crying more and more often. I responded by pouring myself a glass of wine each night after work and sitting outside on the front porch swing.

"You drink too much," Nick would say softly.

"Yeah," I would agree. "You smoke too much," I would add, gazing at the backdrop of the towering mountain range against the kennel across the street.

"I quit smoking," he would sometimes tell me.

"Really?" I'd look at him. "Good," I'd say, truly glad. Then I'd shift my gaze back to the mountains and resume sipping my wine. Nick would go inside without another word, leaving me to finish watching the day end in quiet solitude.

I loosely correlated the crying episodes with my stomachaches, which had also grown more frequent and painful since our first few months in Utah. I stopped mentioning the stomachaches to Nick, having come to accept their routine presence in my life like I did such other immutable factors as dogs licking dinner plates or living in a trailer in Utah. By that time my perspective had shifted from viewing the trailer as a foundation for possibilities to regarding it as a decrepit hovel in which we were trapped. The chances of upgrading our living situation sank lower with each dog Nick added to the kennel. Rather than moving forward, we were settling into our life in that shoebox for the duration of the unforeseeable future.

It never occurred to me to tell my new doctor about the stomachaches, which hadn't subsided since I started my job. Nick would tap on the bathroom door each morning to urge me to hurry.

"Steeeenk," he'd say softly, "I have to go, too."

Sometimes at work the pain would grow so intense that I couldn't keep it all to myself.

"My stomach is killing me," I would say, and whichever coworker I'd confided in would unfailingly place a hand on her stomach.

"Yeah, mine's not feeling so hot today either," she'd say. "There must be a bug going around."

I wondered how everyone managed to live in such constant discomfort, and, eventually, I kept my mouth shut about it. Harmless staples like dry toast, crackers, and chicken noodle soup failed to settle my stomach for any length of time. Causal evidence pointed to the old standby of stress, which also explained the crying.

The pain had never been so constant, and it drained something out of me—an energy or a will. The sicker I grew, the more pieces of my world came apart, and the more pieces of my world that came apart, the sicker I grew. Such was the cyclical nature of anxiety, I supposed, all the while brooding over what I could possibly do about it.

Searching for more gainful employment had led me down a few prospective paths, but nothing panned out in the end. When the job search stalled, I looked into graduate courses only to find none within driving distance. I toyed with the idea of freelancing and concluded it was too big a venture for a lone outsider like myself.

One morning at the office, I overheard Jennifer complaining about the number of clients her husband referred to her for graphic design work. He met a lot of people through his construction business, and as a consequence, she was overwhelmed. Clearly, she needed my help. Buoyed with renewed hope at this foolproof plan, I bided my time until the opportune moment to present my idea of partnering arose.

26

THE SUNDANCE FILM FESTIVAL once again usurped Park City, and this time, I learned firsthand how Heber City locals felt about the event. Not only did my coworkers take extreme measures to avoid the added pageantry of an already pompous city stage, but they urged me to steer clear of the mob scene as well. The problem was, I told them, Nick had to be featured on this TV show—*Wild On* something or other—I wasn't familiar. But other people seemed to know about it. After Nick treated the show's hosts to the grand dog sled tour, he called me at work to tell me they'd invited us to a Sundance party that night. I recognized the sponsors' names, Warner Bros. and VH1, as well as the party's featured band, Everclear.

"You know it's going to be crazy in that town," I said into the phone loud enough for my coworkers to hear.

"Yeah," Nick said. "It'll be awesome."

"Well, I guess we really can't pass it up." I rolled my eyes at Jennifer and shrugged. Clearly, my hands were tied.

The answer to the celebrity riddle was finally within reach. I knew celebrities would grace the otherwise average crowd at the VH1/Warner Bros. party, providing the perfect opportunity to conduct the observational research needed to unravel this enigma. In the Sundance party environment, identifying the qualities that separated celebrities from the rest of the people on earth, I felt positive, would be as easy as finding the flamingo in a grounded flock of Canada geese.

Nick and I drove to the outskirts of Park City and caught a shuttle to Main Street, where we wandered around until it was time to meet his new *Wild On* friends. By the time we reached Harry O's, the site of the festivities, the sidewalk out front resembled a zoo break. The heat emanating from all the animal fur people wore may have kept Nick and I from freezing to death as we merged into the human herd clad in the non-human hides waiting to enter the building. The only coat I owned was a mid-weight Gortex parka that I'd found on clearance at the Eddie Bauer outlet store when we'd first arrived in Utah. Teal had been the only available color, and I felt a bit conspicuous among the more natural hues of the long-haired coats, tasseled leather boots, and coordinated cowboy hats of Sundance Film Festival's elite. It was after 10:00 p.m. Nick had been trying to call the *Wild On* hosts for more than half an hour.

"What were their names again?" I asked. I didn't want to seem rude when we met.

"Brooke Burke and Art Mann," he reminded me for the fourth time just as his phone rang. Pressing the phone to his ear, Nick scanned the area until he saw a hand waving near the front entrance.

"That's her," he said. "Let's go."

We pushed our way through the crowd to the side entrance where Brooke, Art, and entourage were waiting. Forming a cluster, we started toward the door, but a bouncer stopped Nick and I from following the *Wild On* crew into the building. Art yelled from his position at the front of the celebrity pack and, after a few moments of arguing, the bouncer relented. I don't know who Nick and I were supposed to be in relation to the critical *Wild On* team, but our identities didn't matter to the next Harry O's host, who corralled us into a stark, windowless room then disappeared. Nick and I stood off to the side as the cast and crew discussed the situation among themselves. After fifteen minutes, an usher appeared and led us through the party on the main floor, up a set of stairs, and into a second-floor VIP section. A railing separated our section from the rest of the party downstairs, and amphitheater seating descended from the second floor, just beneath the railing, toward the dance floor below. Nick and I waited for the *Wild On* crew to settle in. Then we walked over to the end of the bar where they'd gathered, so I could meet the stars of the show.

Brooke sat on a stool facing in toward the bar, and Art stood behind her with his back against the wall. After introducing me to Art, Nick spent a few moments trying to get Brooke's attention. When he did, she turned halfway toward us on her stool.

"This is my girlfriend, Tara," Nick said. Brooke gingerly extended her hand, allowing her fingertips to graze mine so lightly I wasn't sure it qualified as a handshake.

"It's nice to meet you," I smiled. She may have looked me in the eye for a fraction of a second, but I had never mastered fractions and therefore wasn't familiar with a number small enough to account for the timeframe of the exchange. She turned around to face the bar, leaving me still smiling at the back of her head. After a moment, Nick veered toward an open section of the bar to get us some drinks, and I returned to our previous location at the front of the VIP section, where we'd have a bird's-eye view of the Everclear concert that was already in progress.

Nick wove through the crowd to our previously claimed position holding a bottle of Bass for himself and a clear plastic cup allegedly containing my vodka tonic. I couldn't be sure since neither citrus slice nor sensory evidence of vodka dwelled inside. I sipped the watery mixture and opted out of a second, having also failed to detect bathroom facilities in our region of the VIP area. Another drink might necessitate a trip to the downstairs restroom, at which point I'd surely be discovered as the imposter I was and subsequently returned to the sub-zero sidewalk area, where people much worthier than I still waited to be invited inside.

I'd seen no sign of a coatroom, so my parka dangled over my arm as I watched the crowds and the stage below. "Chemical Smile" blared from the stage, propelling my heart rate toward the pulsing rhythm of the dance floor. A girl in the amphitheater seats, whose loose blonde curls I had admired from behind, turned to face us as she danced. She looked me in the eyes and bared her teeth like a lioness, gyrating and waving her arms to the music. I studied her thickly painted eyes as I sipped my vodka-less tonic and wondered if she was a celebrity I should recognize. There must be celebrities swarming the VIP section, I thought, but they all looked like regular people to me. I wouldn't know a celebrity if I spilled my virgin tonic on one, I realized, and by that point, I wasn't sure I cared.

Nick and I left before the concert was over, anxious to get back to our dogs in the secluded Midway trailer home. We didn't say goodbye to the *Wild On* cast, who had so graciously invited us to the Sundance celebration. As we left, I caught a glimpse of Brooke, bathed in light and besieged by partygoers, smiling now and holding the microphone to her mouth as she bantered with crowds surrounding her and flirted with those amassed by the camera filming her. The light illuminated her magnetic presence, which lured fans like june bugs to the zapper. *She's good at her job,* I realized then, stopping to watch for the briefest of moments before turning toward a different beckoning force—the exit.

That winter, Nick spent significantly more time on his computer than out running sled dogs. Prior to moving from Pennsylvania, I'd questioned my willingness to support a sport like dog mushing. Though I'd never heard reports of cruelty as I had for other dog-related sports, like fighting and greyhound racing, the question lingered until logic effectively suppressed it. *How would I know without firsthand experience?*

I willed myself to try the lifestyle before passing judgment in the same way I'd agreed to try raw onions on a chili dog. Albeit more slowly than the raw onion experience, I learned that dog mushing didn't appeal to me either. I had witnessed no cruelty—at least not from Nick. His dedication to the dogs' welfare likely extended my delusion of acceptance. Still, I could not distinguish the sled dogs from pets.

Katy and Chief lived in our constant company. They ate off our dinner plates, roamed free in the house, and rode in our cars when we traveled. We took them next door to play with the Gardenias' two dogs (Katy's new favorite pastime). Out in the country with all the space in the world, they rarely wore leashes. I couldn't imagine fastening Katy to a six-foot chain and expecting her to spend her life outside. I wouldn't conceive of making her work to prove her worth. She was part of my family.

Try as I may, I found no fundamental difference in the sled dogs. They were friendly and happy and smart. I did not want them to have to work or pull a sled or be crammed into a plywood dog box to ride all the way to heaven knew where Nick might find to run them. But all that was better than being chained to a stake for the better part of most days, which was where they would stay with Nick otherwise occupied. He needed to make money to run the dogs. So I did what I could to help by designing some logo ideas for his "e-commerce" ventures.

Though I still lacked comprehensive knowledge of the business, I fully understood Nick's infatuation with the multimillion dollar sales of single domain names. When the maximum length for domain names increased from seventeen to sixty-four characters, he wanted to buy hundreds of them. He called his friends and family to share his latest stroke of money-making genius. That's when his mother isolated me on the telephone to ask if he was acting manic. I had no idea she'd been watching for signs. The interpretive problem was, Nick often acted in ways that might be considered manic. I construed this behavior as being within the normal boundaries of his extreme personality. From what I understood, he planned to use all the domain names he would purchase for the $20,000 he was going to talk his father into loaning him to build an online shopping network of every service anyone could ever need or want. The idea sounded solid to me, though I vaguely wondered where Nick would find enough time to dedicate to this ambitious venture, given all his dog mushing duties and aspirations. Maybe his mother wondered the same. Nick had been on the phone with her, explaining his plan, when she'd asked to speak with me.

"Go someplace where Nick won't hear you," she'd instructed.

"What's wrong?" I asked.

"How does he seem?" she said.

"Fine, I guess. Like Nick."

"He isn't acting unusual?"

"I'm not sure what you mean," I said.

"Does he seem more hyper than usual, happier, more upbeat?" she prodded.

"Well, yeah. I mean, he's pretty excited about this idea."

"And what do you think of the idea? Does it sound reasonable to you?"

I had no appropriate reference point. I didn't have a millionaire father who bought me cars and took me on helicopter rides and sent me to private schools. I didn't have the ability to think on the financial scale that Nick did.

"Uh, yeah, I guess. I'm not sure how one person could do it all, but he has a bunch of people he works with online. I don't know. I think the idea sounds good."

"O.K.," his mom said then, satisfied with my thirty-second assessment. A few days later, Nick's dad loaned him the money to purchase his pick of domain names in all their hyphenated forms. That's the last I would learn of his online shopping network project.

27

MY PARENTS FLEW IN for their first visit to Utah, and Nick and I treated them to an assortment of scenic mountain drives and Park City tours to expose them to the depth and range of our new home's appeal. We introduced them to the Gardenias and spent time with the sled dogs. Nick took my dad on the first and likely only dog sled ride of his life. By that time Nick had found a trail through the Uinta National Forest, where he trained the dogs twice a week. I'd tag along on a Saturday or Sunday, but most of the training took place during the work week at Strawberry Ridge, approximately thirty miles southeast of our house. From the start of loading the dogs into the truck in Midway to the finish of unloading the dogs back at the kennel, the trip could take upwards of four hours. It wasn't the worst way to spend a Saturday afternoon.

From October through March, pristine snow blanketed miles of land, which ranged in elevation from 8,000 to 9,500 feet. The trail Nick most often traveled wound through the forest where much of the powdery snow was protected from the heating rays of Utah's tenacious sun. The trees lining that trail sometimes parted to reveal breathtaking views of the valley below. When we didn't cross paths with snowmobiles, the silence of the ride transported me into a wonderland reminiscent of fairy tales. Though my mother declined the ride, I couldn't wait to share the experience with my father.

I kneeled between the leaders at the front of the lines, watching my dad struggle to restrain Cinnamon as he clutched the chain around her neck and ran from the truck to the sled, where Nick waited to hook her up with the rest of the team. The usual frenzy ensued, fraught with jumping, howling, and nerve shattering cries that seemed more ghostly that canine. I stepped away from the leaders as Nick released the brake.

"Haaaa—aayke!" he yelled, and the dogs surged forward in concentrated, now silent, effort. As the sled pulled away with my dad in the cargo basket, I closed my eyes to imagine what he must be feeling. My own experiences had felt like gliding on a cloud in heaven by way of sled-dog drawn chariot. The most fascinating part, I noticed after a few rides, was the chain of events that occurred when one of the chariot-pulling dogs relieved him or herself mid-stride. I'd witness these proceedings from my privileged perspective as a passenger in the chariot. Nick would urge the dogs to keep on running, and they'd do just that with barely a blip in the motion as the droppings from one or another bounced off the snow and disappeared behind the sled. The entire display represented a natural wonder from which my fleeting worry about the trajectory of the bounce in relation to my position barely distracted. I was gliding on a cloud in heaven with nary engine sound nor fume. The sporadic puff of fecal odor could not disturb my inner peace. I did not know if Dad would share my fascination with the dogs' secondary talent, but I surmised he'd reach transcendence either way. The gaping grin affixed to his face as they glided into the parking area validated that prediction.

We prepared dinner in the harvest gold kitchen of our rented mobile home the night before my parents were scheduled to fly back to Pennsylvania.

"So how did you like your first trip to Utah?" Nick asked, and I cringed instinctively at the question. I knew my parents had not changed their position on my choice to move with Nick, but I hoped this visit had eased their concerns.

"Park City's great, isn't it?" I said, flashing through the week in my mind to affirm we'd exposed them to the most appealing aspects.

"Sure," my mother said, but I sensed a lack of enthusiasm.

"Well, I'll tell you." My dad picked up his knife and sawed off a portion of pork chop. "Nothing we did compared to the thrill of that dog sled ride," he said, slicing the air with his knife as if to add "and that's final."

In the weeks that followed my parents' visit, an emptiness hung in the trailer air. Nick talked about buying land near Strawberry Ridge and building a house with a dog kennel, so tours could commence from the backyard. I daydreamed about such a home in a remote area of the wilderness with no one around but Nick and the dogs. I mentioned once in casual conversation at work that I enjoyed the company of the sled dogs more than I did most people.

"Well, they don't talk back," Jennifer quipped, leaving me spinning in rapid-reply impotence. As the retaliation window slid shut in my stunned silence, I wondered if she had meant to insult me.

I rarely trumped people's jabs with clever responses. My talent, to my life-long dismay, lay not in snappy comebacks, but in long-term analysis. I pondered the insults people hurled at me long after they'd hit their mark. Jennifer's observation, insult or not, proved to be quite thought provoking.

When Midnight was sick, I had known in an instant. He did not verbalize his feelings, but the message in his demeanor was clear. I felt or otherwise recognized his plea for help. The English language would have served no better in communicating the desperation I sensed. Without words, Midnight spoke to my heart, an epiphany destined to remain subconscious in the absence of Jennifer's remark.

My thought train continued on its tracks to consider the complex communication processes that took place within the canine pack. Sans human intervention, I'd seen the dogs quickly and innately find their positions to form a fully functional team. This amazing feat would not be possible without communication. As I'd never witnessed the formation or experienced the existence of a fully functional human team, it seemed to me that dogs communicated more effectively than people, "talking" notwithstanding.

Having arrived at this triumphant conclusion, I overcame the sting of Jennifer's comment, and shortly thereafter, I approached her with my freelancing idea. She thought it could possibly work, and we invited Lena to meet with us, along with John, the most experienced pre-press specialist in the office. John was so well respected by the company owner that, unlike the rest of the designers and pre-press staff, he handled his own client accounts. He rarely spoke, so I didn't learn of his religious persuasion and status until I'd worked with him for several months. This information came to me by way of eavesdropping on a conversation that ended with Lena asking John if he wore the "holey underwear" and John smirking in lieu of a reply.

"I'm sorry," I said, performing what I hoped they'd interpret as a friendly takeover of their conversation, "but why would anyone wear holey underwear?" I envisioned a one-piece cotton garment hanging in dilapidated rags off someone's body.

"It's a Mormon thing," Lena replied. "John is a steak leader." I briefly wondered what the role of "steak leader" might entail but felt the need to first attend to the holey underwear order of business. *Did the Mormons consider holey underwear to be a sign of humility?* I wondered. *Did they have to wear the same underwear every day, until it became holey?*

"But why does it have to be holey?" I continued after a thoughtful pause.

"I have no idea," Lena said. "It's just what they have to wear. It's supposed to protect them I guess."

"But how would something with holes in it protect anything?" I still didn't get it. Lena burst into laughter.

"No, it isn't holey! It's *holy*—like blessed!" she said.

"Oh!" I laughed to hide my embarrassment and decided, for the moment, to hold all questions about the steak leader position. In time, the art of active listening, as opposed to blatant questioning, would enlighten me to the fact that the term "stake" referred to a division of the church and not, as I had surmised, a juicy slab of beef.

On the rare occasion that John did speak, torrents of print industry knowledge gushed forth as the result of having worked in all possible trenches, from pressman to designer to customer service representative. If we could get John on board, we thought, there was no way our business aspirations could fail. He agreed to come to our first meeting.

As freelancing plans progressed, I missed a few of my weekend kennel visits. I ventured over one Saturday in the late afternoon, and the first thing I noticed was that Sandy had lost her marbles. She darted from corner to crevice with her nose in the stones eating everything "edible" among them she could find, including leftover dog food in all its digested forms. Her inflated abdomen resembled a helium balloon, and if her nose hadn't been glued to the ground in frantic search for food, I may have expected her to float away.

"Nick!" I looked at him in horror. "What's she doing?"

"She's been eating shit."

"Oh my god why?"

"I think she has worms," he said.

"That's not right."

"I know. I have to call the vet and get some worming medicine this week," he said.

I'd seen animals with worms before, but the only time I'd ever seen a dog eat another animal's feces was when Katy had discovered the "gourmet" tidbits that my ex-roommate's cat left in the litterbox. I didn't realize what was happening until Katy had gained more than five pounds (a significant percentage for a dog that normally weighed twenty-six pounds). I returned from work one day and caught her with the culprit hanging out of her mouth. After that disturbing episode and for the benefit of all involved, my roommate raised the litterbox to higher ground. My vet explained that cat food and the resulting feces are loaded with so much protein that dogs can't resist either option.

But Sandy wasn't eating cat food. She was devouring the same dog food she and the other dogs had consumed and digested already. There couldn't be many nutrients at all left in that, I thought, trying to reason beyond my disgust. Sandy was frazzled. She acted like she was starving, and for the first time, she didn't acknowledge my presence in the kennel. I asked Nick about the situation a few days later.

"I wormed her but she's still eating shit," he said.

"Well, you need to take her to the vet."

"I know," he assured me. "I have an appointment this week."

Nick intended to breed some of the kennel dogs once he'd gotten to know his team members, their individual strengths and weaknesses. The mushers he'd worked for in Alaska had gone so far as to freeze the sperm of one of their champions for his future use. Nick planned to use that sperm wisely to build his racing team. His trip to the vet with Sandy altered those plans.

I'd suspected it all along. Sandy didn't have worms. She was pregnant. The accidental breeding must have occurred during one of the many times he'd let the dogs run loose in the kennel. Over the summer, he'd fashioned a corridor out of chicken wire that stretched from the current kennel, across the barnyard, and into the original kennel so the dogs had more room to run. Though he prided himself on knowing when any females were in heat and in separating them from the male dogs when they were, he could not monitor both kennel areas simultaneously. He'd miscalculated Sandy's heat cycle and, as a result, had no idea who the father was.

"It could be any of them," he told me. "Hell, it could be more than one."

"What?" I asked.

"A litter can have more than one father," he said.

"No."

"Yeah. I just talked to the vet about it."

I found myself torn between pure ecstasy at the thought of having puppies and extreme trepidation for their future. Bearing witness to the working lives of full-grown dogs who had likely never experienced anything else had been hard enough. The concept of condemning puppies to such a fate proved borderline unbearable. I conceded that the kennel dogs enjoyed running and even pulling a sled, as Nick often asserted. Some appeared to prefer living outside, and there was no denying that the sled dogs led a more natural life than many species-confused house dogs would ever know. But for once in my life, all those intellectually tangible observations failed to change my perspective: I wanted all those dogs to be house pets. I wanted them to eat off of dinner plates and sneak up on furniture, to sleep in a warm bed and open presents at Christmas. I wanted them to live like Katy and Chief. I vowed to give those puppies as much love and affection as possible—the only resources in my power to give.

Along with impending puppies, my freelancing venture lit the distant horizon with a sunbeam of hope. John had attended only the first meeting, but we kept him informed as discussions progressed. Our biggest decisions revolved around what to purchase based on our designated roles. Jennifer would solicit most of the work, as her husband often identified potential clients through his business. Lena and I would take the lead on production since Jennifer had a young daughter who kept her otherwise occupied. I agreed to invest a few thousand dollars—all the savings I had left from my glamorous Park City job—to purchase equipment. Jennifer would do the same as soon as we determined what type of equipment to purchase.

With plans to remain in our current positions and build the freelancing business over time, we felt no rush to get started. This was my understanding until the day Jennifer approached me at work while I color-corrected a photograph. She looked at me with huge blue eyes that seemed to be holding back the ocean.

"I have to talk to you," she said.

"Sure," I said, trying to read her expression.

"It's John," she continued. "He approached me a couple weeks ago about the freelancing business."

"Oh, cool!" I hadn't heard anything from John on the topic in over a month. I wondered if he'd changed his mind about joining us. "What did he say?"

"He..." she faltered. "He's afraid you're not going to stay in the area."

"What?" I struggled to piece together her meaning.

"He thinks you're going to move back east, if not now, eventually."

"What does that have to—? I don't understand."

"He was already planning to go into business for himself before you and I started talking about it. He asked me to go into business with him instead." As my heart worked on the never-before-attempted feat of skipping three beats at once, I strove to compose my facial expression to appear more understanding than accusing. I didn't have to ask what her response to John had been. It was written all over the ocean threatening to gush from her eyes. "I talked to my husband about it, and he said it's something I can't pass up. I'm so sorry."

"I understand," was all I could say, and I turned back to my screen so she would not see my chin tremble. I braced myself for the extended explanation I expected Jennifer to offer, assuming she'd want to further assuage her own guilt. I kept my focus on the computer screen, concentrating like never before on oversaturating the color levels just enough to give them that eye-catching vibrancy for the newspaper's front page. Jennifer watched me for several more seconds. Then she walked away without another word.

PART IV
A Dream to Follow

28

WHEN I WAS TWENTY-FIVE years old, I made a plan. I had interviewed without success for several positions by that point in time, and regardless of the job field or responsibilities advertised, one question always came up.

"Where do you want to be in five years?" the person conducting the interview would ask, and I'd fumble for a response every time. The constancy of this occurrence led me to believe I was the only college graduate in the free world without a five-year plan. So I promptly made one. By the time I was thirty, I said to myself, I would be gainfully employed in a fulfilling career with abundant opportunities for upward mobility, and I would be deeply committed in an emotionally healthy, long-term relationship with a reasonably flawed (I was realistic, after all) life partner, working together to carve out a bountiful future. Five years represented ample time to accomplish these two life goals, which I felt would lock in the destination coordinates on my highway toward happiness.

The goal seemed so reasonably achievable—like a natural progression in the grand scheme of the universe—that, aside from the brief period at the age of twenty-six during which I'd resigned to my future as a spinster, I never thought to take inventory along the way. Five years after mapping out my five-year plan, I found myself landlocked in a state that may as well have been Mars for all I could relate to anything about it; stranded more than 2,000 miles across the country from my family; stuck in a job with no advancement opportunities in the foreseeable or any other brand of future; entrenched in the dog-mushing dream of a man, I now realized, I hardly knew; and mind-numbingly quickly approaching the age of thirty.

On top of this personal predicament, I'd recently learned that my grammie's health was declining. She'd fallen several times over the course of a few months, and the last fall had sent her to the hospital. She'd since been released, but I could not get it out of my mind.

After dinner one night, I'd so immersed myself in thoughts of how to help Grammie from 2,000 miles away that I startled when Nick spoke beside me on the couch. He said his father planned to bring his new girlfriend for a visit. Based on some email exchanges I'd had with my former coworker Anne, I suspected she had not been apprised of this relatively new relationship. It sounded as if Nick's father had initiated the affair while he and Anne were still dating.

"When is he coming?" I asked, knowing that I couldn't keep it from happening—knowing I shouldn't even be entertaining the thought.

"Next month," Nick said. "They're going to stay here in the trailer."

He answered my next question before it came out of my mouth. His father and guest would stay for a week.

Our visitors arrived during a late winter cold snap, and Nick's father's girlfriend came prepared. She stepped into our ramshackle trailer wearing spiked heel boots and a genuine fur coat. Her frosted nails matched the highlights in her medium-length, stylishly layered hair, not a strand of which had strayed out of place through the six-hour flight from Pennsylvania and subsequent forty-five-minute drive from Salt Lake City. I forced myself to look away from her babydoll nose as we stood in the mud-colored living room making pleasantries. Secretly relieved I'd be working all week while Nick found ways to entertain his guests, I hoped I could concoct enough small talk to navigate amicably through the weekend.

We cooked dinner in the trailer that night, and Nick's father insisted on making dessert. His daughter had given him a recipe that involved baking graham crackers with chocolate and one or two other ingredients. "You won't believe this!" he said as he put the confection together. His excitement over the act of sharing a simple dessert gave him an adolescent air which, I hated to admit, bordered on boyish charm. His button-nosed girlfriend had prepared a beautiful salad bursting with fresh flavor to accompany our dinner, and I found the ice around my heart melting just enough to warn Nick's father about our fickle oven.

It was, undoubtedly, the original oven that came with the trailer, which marked its age at twenty-plus years. Having long since veered from earth's natural space-time continuum, this oven warmed up on its own terms. Preheating required more patience than a person familiar with ovens would be prepared to practice. The absence of an indicator light made determining when the oven had reached the desired temperature like an art form. You just had to get a feel for it. Nick's father, accustomed to cooking in a state-of-the art, restaurant quality oven, was unprepared for the temperament of this appliance. And accepting advice contradicted his nature.

"This oven doesn't work!" he declared five minutes after flipping the dial to 350°. The shrill quality of his voice reminded me of Joe Pesci in the movie *My Cousin Vinny*.

"It works," I said. "It just takes about twenty minutes to preheat."

"Bah," he muttered as he cranked the dial up to 400°. "The temperature's off on this thing."

I considered pointing out that I'd lived in the trailer for more than a year, during which I'd used the oven almost every day. I thought about claiming more knowledge of the oven I'd used almost every day for more than a year than would be possible for him to possess, having just turned it on for the first time ever. Instead, I turned quietly around, walked through the living room, down the hallway, and out the back door to the deck, where I stood inhaling the icy air, counting to ten between breaths to prevent hyperventilating.

I gazed at the network of stars and planets in the clear night sky and thought about the future. My heart rate stabilized with each deliberate breath. I knew that with age, most people morphed into some version of their parents. The longer I lived with Nick, the more similarities I saw between him and his father—the obsession with money and, at times, the voice. My pulse quickened, but before I could work my way into a panic, the back door opened. Nick poked his head out to tell me dessert was ready.

I walked into the smoke-filled kitchen, the odor of burnt chocolate assaulting my senses, and I took my seat at the table. I didn't say a word about the oven, and neither did Nick's father. We ate our charred dessert in relative silence with nothing but the crunch of unnaturally crisp graham crackers connecting us around the dinner table.

I returned home from work on Tuesday afternoon to an empty trailer. Though I knew Nick had taken our guests on a dog sled ride that day, I thought they'd left in the morning. Nick rarely kept the dogs out after dusk, and I'd almost exhausted my powers of rationalizing when I saw the lights of the truck pulling into the kennel. It was dark when they all made it back to the trailer, and I could tell Nick was in no mood to explain. I waited until we were alone in the bedroom to ask what had happened.

"My dad lost his camera out on the ridge," he said. It had been snowing, and Nick knew the odd chance of finding it did not justify the risk of looking. Still, he stopped the team because his father had wanted to search. "He looked for that damn camera for two hours."

"Did he find it?" I asked, half expecting that he did.

"No, he finally gave up because it was getting dark."

"Did you help him look?"

"I couldn't turn the dogs around, and I couldn't leave the team."

"You mean he walked out there on the ridge for two hours by himself in a snowstorm?"

"Yeah," Nick said. "I couldn't stop him."

"Oh my god," I said, thinking about the couple from New England who had gone skiing and never returned to pick up their child at the day care center. Nick knew how dangerous Utah snowstorms could be, especially at an elevation of 8,000-plus feet. Prior to this episode, I'd considered his father to be overconfident, but I hadn't thought of him as careless or disrespectful of nature. Beyond that, he'd put other people in danger.

What an asshole, I thought, and I rolled over and went to sleep.

Earlier that winter, I had developed a dry cough that usually started with a tickle in the back of my throat. Once the cough started, it didn't stop. If I coughed at work, I'd run to the bathroom, which did little to hide my hacking behind the thin door. My coworkers would yell through that door, "Are you O.K.?" In response, I'd cough until I couldn't breathe.

This persistent cough tormented me, waking me several times a night and leaving me terror stricken, convinced I would suffocate in the vast expanse of time it took to draw a breath after each fit. I drained all the air from my lungs every time I coughed. My abdominal muscles perpetually ached, and, through coughing alone, tightened to near washboard condition. Other than the cough, I felt no symptoms of illness, so I waited a month before contacting my doctor. He agreed to see me that day.

Shortly before the receptionist called my name, another patient entered the waiting room exhibiting an audible replica of my cough. I'd been fearful of inciting an uncontrollable coughing fit, should the doctor ask me to demonstrate my symptoms. As I entered his office, I referenced the patient in the waiting area in an effort to thwart the request, but the doctor had no intention of asking me to cough. He'd intuited the source of my torment already and had only to peer down my throat to confirm. Bronchitis, he told me, could be viral or bacterial. He would prescribe some antibiotic pills. If the condition was bacterial, I'd see improvement a few days after starting the medicine. If it was viral, I'd have to wait it out until the virus ran its course.

Nick's father and his girlfriend had arrived on day two of my antibiotic treatment. Though the pills had no effect on my cough, they'd added an element of nausea that magnified with each dose. The night we took Nick's father and his girlfriend to Snake Creek Grill—our favorite local restaurant—I knew a full meal was impossible. I ordered a spinach salad, hoping to make it through dinner without causing an unsightly scene.

"That's all you're getting?" Nick's father said.

"Yes." I replied. "I haven't been feeling well." I thought I heard him snort in response, but with all my energy consumed in quelling my nausea, I could not concern myself with his judgment.

By the time dinner ended, I felt a bit better. *I must have needed food to settle my stomach*, I thought, breathing a sigh of relief as we stood to leave, but the breath caught in my inflamed throat. I suppressed the cough provoked by the telltale tickle, and I followed our party toward the exit door.

Located in the historic railway village of Heber Old Town, Snake Creek Grill connected to the other turn-of-the-century style buildings by wooden plank walkways. As I stepped out the door and onto the first plank, the cough forced its way out, and a full-blown hacking frenzy followed. I stumbled forward as the macerated spinach salad surged up from my stomach and into my throat before ejecting with surprising force and splattering across the pristine planks in a scene rivaling Linda Blaire's projectile display in the original *Exorcist*.

Nick's father and his girlfriend had reached the car. Nick, who had been walking closely behind them, turned to look at me. He stood still for a moment, then proceeded to join his father at the car. I threw up twice more before lifting my head to notice that I was stationed before the restaurant's sizable window. My display had been clearly visible to the roomful of once hungry patrons. I covered my mouth. The restaurant door opened behind me, and I started toward the car without looking back.

"Miss," a voice said, and I walked faster, desperate to disappear into the dusk.

"Miss?" The soft-spoken word echoed in the silence of the empty courtyard. I turned around, my hand still covering my mouth. The restaurant host walked toward me with a glass of water.

"Sorry," I whispered, tears streaming down my cheeks. I watched the man step lightly over the phosphorescent sludge that dripped through the wooden slats of the walkway.

"Are you O.K.?" he asked, holding out the glass.

"I'm fine," my voice cracked. "I'm so sorry." I took the glass.

"It's all right," he said as I took a hurried sip and reached out to return the glass. "No, take it," he said. "You can bring it back later."

"Thank you." I lowered my eyes and rushed to the car.

The next day, I threw the vomit-inducing antibiotic pills into the garbage. Doctors had never helped me as a child, I thought. Apparently they wouldn't help me as an adult either. I promised myself I'd return the glass as soon as I found the courage to enter Snake Creek Grill again. I never did find that courage.

29

MY COWORKERS NOTICED something different about me. I felt them staring for long stretches at a time.

"You look skinny," one of them said, her gaze traversing the length of my body.

"I've been sick," I said, and she shot me a dubious look before walking away.

Lena and Jennifer invited me to lunch and sometimes to dinner or the occasional girls' night out at the bar. As we danced with nameless partners in steel-toed cowboy boots, Wrangler jeans, and belt buckles the size of salad plates, I always wished I were dancing with Nick. Something he'd said bobbed around in my mind, surfacing at odd times like when I danced with a stranger.

Dan and Kelli had invited us over to see the deck they were building off the kitchen of their split-level house. Dan had positioned the steps on the side, but Kelli wanted them to lead into the yard from the middle of the deck. Dan had rearranged the plans to meet Kelli's request.

"The woman of the house makes the rules," he'd shrugged as if referencing a fact of every couple's life.

"That's *crazy!*" Nick had said. "I'd never let that happen." The comment hung in the air for a moment.

"We try to make decisions together," I said, my cheeks burning in response to Dan and Kelli's surprised gaze.

Something about the comment aroused me from whatever stupor I had swaddled myself in. When I agreed to relocate with Nick, I'd accepted him as my life partner. I assumed that he felt the same way. Looking back from the reference point of Kelli's comment and Nick's fervent response, I saw a different reality: two people with discrete lives, so absorbed in their own struggles that no unifying effort had been forged.

I sat beside Nick on the couch one evening after dinner as he watched TV.

"How would you feel about saving some money together," I said, "maybe to buy a house someday?"

"What do you mean?" he replied.

"We could each contribute a couple hundred dollars a month to a house fund, so eventually we can move out of this cardboard shoebox."

"That wouldn't make any sense," he said.

"What part doesn't make sense?"

"A couple hundred dollars a month isn't going to get us anywhere," he said. "We could each contribute a percentage of our income, but that wouldn't be fair because I make so much more money than you."

"So," I paused as the reality sank in. Nick had no intention of saving for our future. "You don't even think it's worth trying?"

Memories crashed like a tidal wave in my mind. "Well, you just haven't met the right man yet," the Gardenia's mystery friend had declared. Whitney Houston's version of "I Will Always Love You" grew into a class 5 hurricane in my head—

"Nope," Nick said. "That makes no sense at all."

The next time we visited the Gardenias, we saw that they'd built a small landing off the front of the new deck in preparation for stairs that would lead from the second floor to the ground. The stairs, they explained, would attach to the right side of the landing, which is why that side had no railing. We each grabbed a bottle of beer and walked out to the deck, which Dan and his brothers had constructed over the past few weekends.

"Go out to the landing," Dan said from behind me, and I sidled up to the front railing. I felt an abrupt jerk and found myself still standing on the landing about six feet lower than its original position. Another violent jolt, and I was standing on the ground, legs between the railing slats, knees slightly bent in dismount position. Dan stood beside me on the right. In my left hand, I still held my bottle of beer. I looked at Dan.

"Are you O.K.?" he said.

"I think so," I was still standing between the slats. "Are you?"

"Yeah," he said, stepping over the railing. I bent and straightened my knees to make sure everything was intact and functional, then gingerly lifted one leg at a time over the railing.

"Are you two O.K.?" Nick called from the deck above, and Dan told him that we were. I looked at the bottle in my hand.

"I didn't even spill my beer," I called up to Nick who let out a half-hearted laugh.

"What happened?" I said to Dan.

"We didn't have time to cement the porch legs in, and the ground must have been soft from the rain we had last week. The support beams slipped into the holes we dug for the cement."

"I had no idea what was going on," I said. "I felt two jerks and then I was standing on the ground."

"It's a good thing I moved," he said.

"What do you mean?"

"I was standing right behind you. I stepped around you to the railing as soon as I felt the porch move." I looked at him. "I would have crushed you," he said.

Over the past eighteen months, Nick had attended conferences in Florida, Las Vegas, New Orleans, and London for his Internet business. He'd return from each event with a more explicit account of conference activities. After returning from a recent trip, he described, in more detail than I deemed necessary, his experience and feelings after "dropping X." I must have looked shocked.

"Well I can tell you this," he said, looking into my eyes. "I turned down a lap dance for you." He smiled and touched my cheek.

Nick's conference stories had sparked a dim light of suspicion deep within the forest of my memory. As he returned from each of those conferences with more lucid descriptions, the suspicion illuminated into a spotlight that searched for something hidden in the shadows. The fact that Nick shared all these stories meant he had nothing to hide, I'd successfully assured myself until lap dances entered the picture. But his lap dance denial drew the searching spotlight to its target—my own denial. Like a deer caught in that spotlight, the truth had nowhere left to hide.

The "adult" portion of Nick's past venture and his current website ranking business, I now realized, had always been one and the same. Questions I'd never allowed myself to consider now boiled to the surface, and I summoned all my courage to vocalize them.

"Those parties you go to at conferences sound pretty crazy," I said one night after dinner.

"Yeah," he said. "You have no idea."

"Why are they like that?"

"It's just part of the business. That's what those guys do," he said preoccupied by the television.

"What guys?" I asked, knowing nothing but the first names of a few people in his network of Internet peers.

"You know," he said, and he looked at me with a hint of confusion. "The guys I always go with. The ones I work with."

"Nick," I said. "I don't even know what you do." He turned to face me directly.

"I've told you what I do."

"It's still pornography, isn't it?" I looked down at the couch.

"It's website promotion," he said, "and what we do isn't illegal."

"I thought you got out of that after we moved here."

"Tara, it's the only way I can make enough money to be here—to have the dogs. That business was bringing in more than ten grand a month just a little while ago."

I knew his business had been successful, but I had no idea of the extent. Nick had spent all that money, and more, by the time he told me about it.

"So, it isn't going to stop."

"It's my work. It's what I do," he said.

The deflated and ill feeling I'd fought off so long ago, now sank in to stay. I stood and walked back to the bedroom.

Anymore, when I smiled, it didn't feel like I was smiling. I hoped nobody noticed because I had no words to explain. I'd find a hiding place and go there to cry on a daily basis. Or I'd cry right out in the open if I thought no one was looking. I wondered if a person's brain chemistry could be permanently changed by long periods of depression. *If a person cried every day for say, two years, would she ever be able to pull herself out of the pattern? Could the loss of hope take up permanent residence after squatting so long in one's mind, body, and soul?*

I stopped bothering to question what had transpired in the universe to render every decision I had made and every event that took place over the past several years so misguided and doomed. From my car breaking down to my computer breaking down to Nick's Jeep breaking down to my body breaking down to losing my glamorous Park City job to my latest failure at freelancing—my parents had been right. We were just unlucky.

"Life's not fair," my mother always said.

Oh my heck, I thought now, *she wasn't kidding.*

I stopped belting out songs on my way to work and thought instead about whistling. Not once since I'd moved to Utah had I been able to whistle. I'd tried drinking more water and even dampening my lips, but all I could muster was the hollow whoosh of a light wind moving through a dried up wheat field. I'd had to invent a new call for Katy, who was used to my whistling back in Pennsylvania, because the sound of wind through a dried up field was all too common where we now lived.

My thirtieth birthday found me depleted of energy, options, and hope. It was Friday the 13th, April 2001, and I told Nick we needed to talk.

"Nothing's working out for me here," I said. Nick sat perched on the river rock wall between the living room and kitchen.

"I know," he said.

"I don't feel like we have a future. I don't like my job, and I have no options here."

"I know," he said again, linking and unlinking his fingers as he studied the dirt-colored carpet.

"I think I should move back home," I said finally, and he looked at me. Tears trickled down his cheeks.

"I know that's the best thing for you," he said. Now I turned to look at the carpet and the tears welled up in my own eyes.

We agreed to split all the furnishings we'd purchased together, based on each other's needs. I told him I wanted to stay through the summer to help with the puppies. I knew I would never be back—not while Nick was still here—not while the sled dogs I'd grown so attached to remained in the kennel. I could not abandon everyone I loved so abruptly.

I'd never felt so sick in my life. I was thinner than I had ever been. My genetically bountiful Italian inner thighs had diminished to the point where they no longer rubbed together when I walked (a condition my mother taught me to refer to as "chub rub"). I'd had those thighs since puberty. Though I wasn't complaining about my newfound miniature physique, it didn't seem like my own body. I'd come to terms, over the past two years, with dropping from a size 6 to a 4 and then to a 2, but when my pant-size dwindled down to 0, I did worry just a little.

I blamed my health problems on the barrage of unfortunate circumstances that had besieged me over the past several years—since before moving to Utah and even prior to meeting Nick. I'd tried so hard to achieve success in my jobs, in my relationship, in my life, but no matter how hard I worked, the success I sought eluded me. And no matter how intensely I reasoned, I couldn't figure out why.

I started out as an overachiever, I thought. What had happened to change that? What in my basic personality had shifted, and where in my life had I gone wrong? I still felt like the same person, albeit much smaller now. I still put forth the same amount of effort to succeed—probably more so. Why, time after time, did I fail?

I blamed the people around me. I blamed Utah. I blamed the whole wide world. I'd changed as much about myself as I could change in attempt to fit in, but Utah had proceeded to chew me up before spitting me out. I could not survive in such barren conditions, I thought, noting everything external as a source of my decline. Stressful conditions caused anxiety, I knew for a fact, and anxiety made people sick. My grammie suffered. My mother suffered. Now I suffered too.

I did not consider an alternative—that my problems might stem from something broken inside, struggling to find its way out. I never looked inward for answers, where the truth had been simmering for years. It would boil to the surface with or without my consent. I never could do things the easy way.

30

I HAD EVERYONE AT WORK on high alert for puppy arrival, which could be any day. Sandy looked like she had swallowed a beach ball. Based on the interest they'd always shown in the baskets of kittens and other critters brought in by their staff, I assumed the family who owned the publishing company would respect the significance of my first litter of puppies. When Nick called the office on a Friday afternoon to tell me Sandy was in labor and had already given birth to her third puppy, I jumped out of my chair and ran in circles repeating, "The puppies are coming!" before sprinting to the time clock and yelling in the direction of the raised eyebrows behind me as I flew out the door, "I have to go! The puppies are coming!"

I arrived at the kennel as Sandy gave birth to her fifth puppy, and she showed no signs of slowing down. Nick, who had been monitoring the proceedings for several hours, relinquished his post to look for a cardboard box so he could transport the puppies across the street. They'd live in the shelter of our garage with Sandy until they were weaned and old enough to move into the kennel. He'd purchased a plastic kiddy pool for their enclosure and lined it with blankets for warmth. The pool awaited their arrival in the garage that day as I sat before Sandy, mesmerized by the surprisingly gory show. Her instincts served well as puppies continued to emerge. When Nick returned with the box, she was up to number eight.

"Isn't she done yet?" he asked.

"Apparently not," I said.

"Oh my god!" he laughed, and I realized he'd just gained an entire team of sled dogs.

"Poor Sandy," I said. Her eyes had assumed a wild cast, desperate as she was to finish this job. With her snout saturated in blood, she struggled to clean the puppies that pushed forth with each contraction. Nick and I stared at the untouched sac beside her, trying to determine if it was a puppy or afterbirth. When she got around to working on it, the sac revealed a puppy.

"Do you think they'll all survive?" I asked, worried for the first time since Nick had told me about the pregnancy.

"I doubt it," Nick said. "I've never seen a dog have this many puppies. She probably won't have enough nipples to feed them all."

"You can do it, Sandy," I said to her quietly. She looked at me with a vacant gaze and continued her work. Tiny wet puppies of various colors squirmed around her. At last, she hit the magic number and was finished.

We sat in silence as she stretched out to feed all ten of her offspring. They looked like piglets with their eyes sealed shut and their ears barely perceptible on their heads. They inched forward on round bellies with rubbery legs paddling toward their mother. My heart nearly broke at the scene, and it looked, by some miracle, as if all ten puppies were feeding.

"Nick," I said, craning my neck toward the puppies, "I think they all found a nipple!" He leaned above Sandy and reached in to separate the puppies.

"Wow," he said. "She's got that crazy long torso."

"Do you think she can do it?" I looked at him.

"We'll have to wait and see, sweetie." Sandy lifted her head at the sound of our voices, her eyes now steady and clear. She shifted her gaze from Nick to me then lay her head back down with a sigh. Nick put his arm around my waist, and I rested my head on his shoulder as we watched his new sled team nurse.

Our time together was ending, but that fact hadn't doused my feelings. Nick and the sled dogs were my family in Utah. Over two years, the roots around them had grown thick and tangled, and I didn't want to cut them loose. So I let myself feel the love I still had. I gave myself that small freedom. It would all be over naturally soon enough.

With the horizon hidden in the fog of my unknown future, I focused on the daily light of ten perfect puppies. Puppy therapy, I called the hours I spent each day after work, sitting with them in the garage until the sun went down.

When they were five weeks old, we carried the puppies into the backyard to romp and wrestle and climb all over us, piercing our skin with their razor-sharp toenails and licking our faces with their buttermilk puppy breath. A few weeks later, Nick took them on their first "puppy walk." We opened the fence gate, and they followed us into the field behind the house. "Puppies, puppies, puppies!" we called, in the same way we'd beckoned since they were old enough to squirm in our direction. All ten puppies came to terms with their running legs, bouncing into each other, falling down, and getting lost in the weeds that were taller than they were. Nick soon identified the fast puppies and those who lagged behind. A few weeks later, we drove them to Strawberry Ridge where they ran behind Nick on his mountain bike because, in that short time, the puppies had outpaced us on our walks.

As summer progressed, I solidified plans for my departure. My dad would fly to Utah in late August. We'd rent a U-Haul, and he'd help me finish packing. Then we'd drive the 2,000 miles to Pennsylvania together. I'd already applied for several jobs back east, one of which, had I not known better, seemed to be designed just for me. The position was in public relations at Lock Haven University where my father had taught for thirty-three years. I'd graduated from LHU's communications department magna cum laude and had worked as an intern in the same PR department one summer.

After a somewhat shaky phone interview, the university flew me in to meet, face-to-face, with representatives from four levels of the organizational hierarchy. I felt at home with members of the interview committee I'd previously known as students of my father. One had been my childhood babysitter. The interview culminated in a conversation with the university president, and by the time I flew back to Utah, I felt hopeful, if not confident in my chances of obtaining the position. It seemed, for the first time in two years, like I'd finally stumbled onto the right track.

A couple weeks before I was scheduled to move, Nick went to another conference. He hired a neighbor to care for the kennel dogs, and I volunteered to look after the puppies. Just shy of three months old, they now had free reign of the fenced-in backyard. I knew the routine. Feed in the morning, then at noon, then in the evening. Water after feeding. Shovel after everything.

The Friday Nick left, the Gardenias invited me to a party at their house. Shortly after my third shot of tequila, I asked Dan's brother, who was a practicing Mormon and who, accordingly, was not drinking tequila with the rest of us, about the Mormon belief system. I had been living in Utah surrounded by the Mormon religion and culture for almost two years, and all I knew were a few facts about their undergarments and exorbitant Jell-O consumption (which I'd learned was a dietary staple due to the cost-effective nature of the item in relation to the number of children they tended to produce—a number which, I'd also heard, was much higher than the national average). The Mormons performed mystical feats with Jell-O, I could attest from the few picnics our landlord and her family had invited us to. I'd once heard a rumor of scrambled egg Jell-O, but the notion was so absurd I chalked it up as urban Mormon legend, having never personally witnessed the dish in its (reconstituted) flesh. With my curiosity stoked by alcohol, the time seemed right to learn more about this religion and its effect on the culture before I left the state forever.

"So, Mark," I said as I moved toward him. "What do the Mormon people believe in?"

"Oh," Dan stepped in front of Mark. "You don't want to know," he said.

"No, I do," I said. "I'm really interested in different belief systems." Mark poked his head around Dan's mountainous frame.

"Trust me," Dan said as Mark opened his mouth to speak, "you don't want to know this."

"What doesn't she want to know?" Kelli yelled over the music from behind the bar.

"She asked Mark about the Mormon religion," Dan answered.

"No!" Kelli bellowed in response. "That is not something you want to ask."

"Why not? I really want to know. I'm curious about different religions." *What the hell is wrong with these people?* I wondered. *Do Mormons sacrifice babies?*

"Girl," Kelli responded, "get over here and do another shot."

I woke up the day after the Gardenias' party feeling like my head had spent the night in a pressure cooker. I'd expected the nausea that consistently set in after a night of drinking tequila—a requirement at the Gardenias' parties. But on this morning after, I had ten puppies to feed, water, and clean up after. I managed to dish out the food, making the puppies wait to eat until I said it was O.K. as Nick, for some reason, had taught them. When I walked back inside to the kitchen, I heard someone knocking at the front door. I peered through the kitchen window to see Dan's brother, Mark, standing on the front porch. Before I could concoct a strategy for watering the puppies without being spotted, Mark glanced to his right and saw me staring at him through the window. He waved. I placed the water bowls on the counter and opened the door.

"I'm filling up water bowls for the puppies," I said, standing in the doorway and hoping Mark would catch the hint that I was in no disposition to entertain a visitor. He looked at me in silence until I finally stepped aside. "Come on in if you want to," I said. He followed me to the sink. "What's up?" I held one of the large rubber bowls under the spigot.

"You said you wanted to know more about the Mormon religion, so I thought I'd stop by and talk to you about it."

What had seemed like a good idea in the middle of a party after three shots of tequila now seemed more like torture in the middle of a hangover with ten hyper puppies to care for.

"Oh," I said turning off the water and preparing myself for the very speech I'd feared prior to my move two years earlier.

Mark said something about the time in history when Jesus was alive, referencing, if my ears did not deceive me, a Jesus-equivalent living in America during that same period. As I processed his words, a flash outside the kitchen window caught my eye. I moved in for a closer look and saw a puppy, free as daylight, running in the open yard. Another puppy appeared, and then another. "Oh no, the puppies are out," I muttered as Mark continued his speech. "I'm sorry," I said, lunging for the door as the realization sank in. "I have to go!"

The puppies had escaped once before by digging a tunnel under the trailer from the fenced-in yard to the freedom of the side yard. Nick had solved the problem by blocking the opening with large rocks from a leftover pile that Dan had not yet moved into his new yard. The puppies had remembered their original escape route. Now stronger, they'd moved some of the rocks and reopened the tunnel to freedom.

I leapt from the porch into the yard, making sure the puppies saw me. Then I invoked the call Nick and I had used on puppy walks, bike rides, and every time we were with them, which was every day, multiple times a day.

"Puppies puppies puppies!" I shouted, and they stopped in their tracks. I crouched in that split second of eye contact, then I turned and ran away from them. They took immediate chase, following me in a wide circle through the yard and toward the trailer porch, where Mark now stood looking somewhat lost. I brushed past him through the door and into the trailer, puppies in proper tow until they reached the doorway. Rather than entering the trailer, they stopped for a moment, then ran in circles around the porch. As I scrambled to corral the puppies into the house, I dutifully apologized to Mark for lacking the time to continue our Mormon conversation, and he seemed relieved enough to take his cue and leave.

After eyeballing the mountain of massive rocks and calculating the measures required to ensure that the rest of the puppies did not push their way through the reopened tunnel, I was now sorry I'd sent Mark away. I dragged several boulders, each of which I was sure amounted to half my body weight, across the yard to the mouth of the tunnel. When absolutely certain the escape route was secure, I returned the three rogue explorers to the fenced yard. It was 10:00 a.m., and I collapsed back into bed.

The rocks held up for the rest of the week, but I made no resistance when the time came to relinquish puppy duty upon Nick's return. The puppies, I learned through this trial, had outgrown my caretaking abilities. They'd sprouted so quickly that I was sure they would mutate, at any moment, from adorable toddlers to awkward teenagers. They showed signs already with their mismatched ears and knobby knees. They were getting too large to pick up and cuddle. It wouldn't be long before they turned into dogs, at which point, their working lives would begin. My role as the nurturer, for whatever difference it had made, was coming to an end. These puppies belonged to Nick, as did all the sled dogs, and nothing I could do would change that. Nick had big plans for his team. The puppies' transition had already begun.

At various stages in the puppies' development, Nick had walked each of the sled dogs over from the kennel to the backyard to meet them. When the puppies were almost three months old, he used the truck to transport them to the kennel where they ran, supervised by us, with the big dogs still tethered to their chains. The puppies frolicked like teenagers, taunting the big dogs then flopping over to expose their bellies. Giant tongues lolled out of their mouths as they gamboled in the kennel, taking full advantage of their free range. The sled dogs played dutifully, exhibiting laudable patience for the juvenile behavior to which they'd been subjected. That's when I knew the puppies were going to be O.K. What I didn't know was how everything would work out for my old friend Jax. I still felt a connection with the dog I'd kept company as he recovered from his scuffle with Rocky so long ago, but Nick had never warmed up to him.

"He doesn't pull," Nick would tell me when I questioned his lack of faith in Jax's ability. It looked to me like Jax pulled as much as the other dogs, but I wasn't the one measuring.

Things have a way of working out, I told myself on the day Nick transferred the puppies to the kennel for the last time. I said goodbye to the puppies and to all the dogs who comprised my extended family in Utah. I devoted extra attention to Jax.

"Promise me you won't sell him," I said to Nick as I rubbed Jax's snow-white face and looked into his ice-blue eyes.

"Sweetie, I can't promise you that," Nick said. "I don't even think anyone would pay for him!" He threw his head back and laughed.

"Please," I said. "He deserves to have a good life. He fits in here." I burst into tears.

"O.K., O.K.," Nick put his arms around me and rubbed my back as I sobbed into his shoulder. "I'll try," was all I could get him to promise.

Though I told her repeatedly I didn't need help, Lena's instinct for a friend in need outweighed my resolve to pretend I didn't fit that description. She showed up the day after my dad flew in, prior to which I hadn't packed a single box. Lena tore through the trailer like a wrapping, packing, taping, labeling cyclone. I think I helped.

Nick hung around as we packed, periodically retiring to his office or the bedroom or out to the backyard. When we crossed paths in the narrow hallway between the living room and the bedroom, we didn't look at each other. We hugged, and we cried. But we didn't look.

I'm abandoning him, I thought. Visions of Nick all alone in the trailer—all alone in the whole state of Utah—haunted me, and I pushed subsequent thoughts of the sled dogs and puppies out of my mind. Something awful hung in the air. If Lena hadn't been there with her mission that was my mission but that I couldn't carry out—if she hadn't arrived with her son to play with Katy as we worked through the day or to laugh her cherub's laugh...

But she was there. We finished packing the fifteen-foot rental truck my dad and I had picked up in Salt Lake City the day before. Equipped with a car trailer, the truck would carry all my belongings, including Betty Blue, back home. I took the couch. Nick got the bed. I took the dishes and pots and pans we'd purchased together, and Nick kept those we'd brought with us from Pennsylvania. We each took a handmade bookshelf. He still had his futon along with one of the computer desks and one of the dressers we'd bought together. I took their twins. We were even.

Dad treated everyone to dinner, and we spent one last night in the trailer. I said goodbye to Nick at seven o'clock the next morning. One more hug. No more tears. I never went back to the kennel.

My cough loosened up shortly after my dad and I got on the road. Though I sounded much worse with a chest full of congestion, this new cough ended in relief rather than in convulsive fits that left me gasping for air. Physically, I felt better than I had in months. Dad and I took turns driving as Katy curled herself into the narrow space between the two seats in the cab. Accustomed as she was by this time to traveling in a variety of conditions, she knew to fall asleep and stay that way for most of the two-and-a-half-day trip.

I asked about Grammie, but Dad didn't have any new information. We talked about my job search and whether or not he'd heard anything from Lock Haven University since my interview. He hadn't. Most of the trip passed in silence with me lost in my thoughts and Dad not knowing quite what to say. I didn't have the words to explain what had happened. I thought about my girlfriends who, over the years, I'd judged harshly for changing to accommodate their partners. I never thought it could happen to me. But in four years with Nick, I'd sunk so deeply into relationship compromise mode that I now emerged on the other side unable to recognize myself. I wondered if I'd ever get to know—let alone like and respect—this person I'd become. At the moment, I couldn't be certain of anything.

We stayed overnight in Nebraska and then in Ohio, and when we hit Pennsylvania, I didn't need a welcome sign to tell me I was home. The trees that lined Route 80 leaned over the road, reaching toward the truck and exhaling their oxygen through the vents and into my lungs. I breathed it in with greed, then coughed and rolled down the window. A warm breeze flowed through the cab. A hint of musk hung in the base notes that danced in the dense air. *Water*, I thought, *life. Lush green, nurturing trees—thick forests rich with nourishing soil.* I closed my eyes and took another deep breath—*I am home.* I opened my eyes and exhaled the rich, Pennsylvania air. *This is the beginning,* I thought, *all over again.* I wondered if I'd be able to whistle now that I was home. Just then, I didn't have the motivation to try. *It can only get better from here,* I told myself, and then it hit me. I'd left Utah without completing my self-assigned mission. I never uncovered the mystery of the lower-alcohol-content beer.

31

I REGAINED EVERY POUND I'd lost during my six-month battle with bronchitis, and I put on a few extras in the process. Living with my parents after twelve years of independence provided a life-sustaining safety cushion which, in spite of my gratitude, felt like a natural abomination. *What kind of a person requires rescuing by her parents at the age of thirty?* I asked myself repeatedly. *A failure,* was my sole response.

Just when I thought I'd reached the lowest point in my life, the call came to inform me that I had not been selected for the public relations position at my alma mater. I could not help but wonder what cosmic anomaly had transpired to rob me of my rights, not only to the position that had seemed like my destiny, but to any prospects for well-being whatsoever? In a show of empathy, a few members of the hiring committee invited me to lunch after the news was delivered. I joined them to salvage my pride, but the lunches I looked most forward to were those each Tuesday with Grammie and Aunt Janet. I'd adopted their established routine as a means of escape from the reality of all my failures. The time I spent with Aunt Janet and Grammie stood outside the boundaries of worldly expectations.

"It's the university's loss," they contended, and I knew, whether or not I agreed, they believed it.

Three months after moving back to Pennsylvania, still jobless and domestically dependent, I saw a sign. Upon returning to the area, I'd spotted a house located ten miles from my hometown. It was small and cottage-like with pale yellow siding—charming and perfect for Katy and me. Each time I passed it, I hoped we'd someday live in such a home. The day I saw the "For Rent" sign in the front yard of that little yellow house, I pulled into the driveway to write down the phone number.

With confidence in nothing but the desperation I felt to revive some semblance of independence, I moved out of my parents' home before any prospects for income solidified. I used the savings from my job at the real estate company, never having spent it on freelancing equipment, for the first month's rent and security deposit. A week after Katy and I moved into our three-room home, I received a job offer for a web design position at a company thirty-five miles away.

The drawback to having a job was the time it detracted from my helping Grammie. She'd been battling an infection in her big toe that had started with a sore caused by a rock in her shoe. The wound had since developed into a sizeable abscess. As a diabetic, she was in danger of losing the toe. I'd sometimes drive Grammie to her appointments (on time, now that Nick had instilled the importance), happy to finally do something useful.

Sitting in the podiatrist's waiting room, I'd marvel at the decorations on the office walls. The most fascinating work of art, by my estimation, was the framed macramé bare foot, which looked to have been severed at the ankle. Every once in a while the doctor would call me into the examining room as a witness while he scolded Grammie in frustration at finding coarse black hairs in her socks and around her bandages. He'd command me to watch as he fished one of the offending hairs out of the deep cavity in her toe using a set of absurdly long tweezers that looked like a medieval instrument of torture.

"This is what's making it so difficult," he'd say to me, shaking the tweezers in front of my face. "She has got to stop letting that dog of hers sleep under the covers!"

I'd promise to talk some sense into my grammie while shooting her the mock evil eye for getting me in trouble, too. She'd respond with a shrug of sheer innocence, and we'd both stifle the impulse to laugh at the fuming foot doctor still waving his terrifying extraction tool.

After each appointment, we'd feast on whatever food struck our fancy that afternoon, most often Pizza Hut pan pizza.

Starting the new job limited my time with Grammie, and getting sick a month later eradicated that time altogether. The symptoms were similar to my standard brand of anxiety-induced trauma, but the Gatorade treatment had no effect this time. I was at my parents' house on Christmas day when a couple of their friends stopped in to visit. Noting my unusual lack of enthusiasm for party food, they told me about a stomach virus that was going around. Everyone seemed to have it, they said, and it usually lasted a week or two.

Another week passed, but the virus remained, draining my strength to the point of exhaustion. I scarcely had energy to walk from one room to the next in my tiny house. I appealed to my dad to help me walk Katy, which he did as often as possible. After about three weeks, desperation propelled me to the emergency room. The attendant tested my blood pressure while I was sitting and again while I was standing, then he hastened to start an IV. Not only was I severely dehydrated, he told me, but my potassium levels were much too low.

In less than an hour, I cultivated a whole new respect for hydration. I no longer felt dizzy or gasped for breath from the overexertion of standing, and I could walk more than five steps without stopping to rest. I felt like a new person, and I celebrated by feasting on a comfort meal of roast beef with gravy over fluffy white bread. The past few weeks of illness had reduced my diet down to saltine crackers and chicken noodle soup. As I sopped up the succulent gravy with soft, springy bread, my fork full of tender roast beef, I knew I'd finally kicked that stomach virus. But my confidence was short-lived. That night, almost as quickly as the IV fluids had pumped up my energy, the stomach virus purged it back out.

With all the strength I had left, I continued driving the thirty-five miles to and from my new job. From August through November I had applied for every position I'd seen advertised in the state of Pennsylvania with a description that resembled my qualifications. I'd received only one offer—the one I took—and I hauled my decrepit body to precious work every single day.

The week after I'd been to the emergency room, a coworker offered to run out for bagels. I knew it was risky, but with my illness continually purging all nutrients from my body, it felt like I hadn't eaten in a month. Against that primal hunger, common sense stood no chance.

Ten seconds after devouring half a bagel, the nausea came in a dizzying wave. It was 11:00 a.m., and I had to leave work. I called in sick the next day, and the day after that. I'd run out of ideas for fighting this illness and suspected that, if I didn't seek help soon, the next thing I'd run out of would be time. I called the family friend who'd prescribed the iron supplements in lieu of a blood transfusion so many years ago—the doctor I'd renounced when the supplements failed. He agreed to see me that week.

My dad drove me to the appointment. He helped me out of the car and supported me by the arm across the parking lot, up four steps, and into the office. I sank into the first chair I came to in the waiting room, breathing heavily from the effort of walking what amounted to less than twenty feet. I could not imagine what was wrong with me, but I had hope that the doctor could help.

In the examining room I said, "I feel like I'm dying." The doctor asked me how many times a day I was going to the bathroom and if it seemed like I was eliminating more than I was taking in.

"About ten," I said, "and I have no idea." He didn't ask if I'd ever experienced anything similar, but he did tell me there had been a stomach virus going around for a few weeks.

He concluded, "I think you're getting better," and he smiled.

That's when I lost hope.

32

MY MOTHER FOUND ME crumpled and helpless on the bathroom floor of my little yellow house. I had been ill for seventeen days. She'd stopped by earlier that morning but, for reasons I had not the will to wonder about, had left abruptly. She would later tell me that she'd seen in my eyes a look she had seen only twice before in her life—once in my great-aunt's eyes days before she passed away, and once in my great-grandfather's eyes, also shortly before he died.

She drove straight to the doctor's office where she marched through the waiting area, burst through the doors to the nurses' station, and stood with tears streaming down her cheeks as she commanded the doctor to help her daughter or find someone else who would. The doctor did not argue, and my mother returned to escort me back to the emergency room.

Several nurses in the ER tried to insert an IV before calling an EMT who, they must have known, would not accept failure as an option. He found success after several moments by twisting the needle in a variety of directions under the skin and jabbing repeatedly until it penetrated a vein I hadn't previously known existed in the base of my left thumb.

I learned that the hospital had no beds available or, rather, not enough staff to accommodate new patients in the available beds. So I remained on the metal folding cart in the ER overnight. Every few hours, a different doctor came to check on me. One of them looked at my fingernails and asked how long they'd been curled over the tips of my fingers like that. "Forever," I told him, "but they've gotten worse in the past couple of years."

In the morning, my mother filled out the admittance paperwork and a nurse wheeled me into a hospital room with a real mattress and a bathroom, seemingly, for my use alone. Under normal circumstances, having a bathroom to myself would have brightened my spirits, but by that time, I had no spirits left to brighten. My life was out of my hands, and all I could do was watch from the fringes as the world proceeded at warp speed around me.

One week earlier, my doctor had told me with all the confidence I'd ever seen in a human being that I was on the mend from the terrible stomach virus that had been going around. I was "definitely getting better," he'd said in his private office that day. Upon first visit to my hospital room, the same doctor declared my potassium levels to be dangerously low—among the lowest he'd ever seen.

Until that time, I'd endured the multiple IV stab wounds and a new puncture wound inflicted every six hours for the purpose of extracting blood, but the potassium turned my IV solution into liquid fire. As the scorching pain extended into the flesh of my wrist and traveled up my arm, I felt the familiar warmth of tears on my cheeks. For two years, those tears had been my most constant companions.

I must have flinched when my doctor ordered another potassium drip several days later. When I told him that it hurt, he adjusted the ratio so it didn't damage my veins. "It shouldn't hurt," he said quietly. The same doctor who, the previous week, had told me with a self-assured smile that I was getting better now looked at me with a curious tilt of his head. I tried to define the look in his eyes, but desperation did not capture it. Though his face was a picture of professionalism, his eyes, if mine did not deceive me, held something akin to sorrow.

Every day he called a specialist with an update on my condition. Every day the specialist told him about the stomach virus that was going around. Courtesy of the IV, I'd gained the requisite level of hydration to once again recognize my face in the mirror, but I continued to eliminate more than I ingested. This I knew, because they measured. At one point I wondered what remained in my body to eliminate, but the images this conjured proved unbearable in my given state. I quickly banished the thoughts.

Instead, I considered the concept of dignity. Though I knew chances were likely that I'd experienced dignity once, maybe even possessed or enjoyed it, that state of existence was so far gone—years since removed—I could no longer remember how it felt. Hospitals don't allow for dignity, anyway. That's a life lesson learned the moment you trade all your undergarments for an approximate square yard of hospital-blue, threadbare fabric masquerading as a backless gown. At this pinnacle, dignity transforms from an illusion of superiority into a cruel joke on all humanity. (And if that isn't enough, the subsequent measuring of bodily eliminations will step right up to hammer the last nail in dignity's coffin.)

Who invented this circular concept that is destined to turn with venomous disdain on each and every one of us some day? That's what I wanted to know. Luckily, much of my dignity had sidled off long before the hospital experience. Imagine the damage potential in one who is not so fortunate. A person, I considered, who does not experience dignity-crushing events at a still formative age may never learn that having dignity is the ultimate exercise in self-deception. At least I'd figured this out before it was too late. That I'd once had dignity was now the impossible concept to grasp. This is how comprehensively it vanishes. Before the hospital, I realized, I'd been trying to recapture my dignity. In the hospital, by contrast, dignity was not an option.

How freeing, I thought as I lay in the hospital bed awaiting the daily measurement of my excreta.

We developed a routine. After talking to the doctor each morning, my mother called my employers to tell them I would need to stay in the hospital for another day. Then we watched *The View*. My father visited several times a day and paced the floor until he had to return to work. One morning the nurse asked if I wanted to see the chaplain or to have my hospital announcement in the local newspaper. *No, and are you kidding?*

Nevertheless, the chaplain stopped by on one of my less fortunate days. I was resting in mid-afternoon with the bed completely reclined when a man poked his head through the doorway.

"Tara," he said.

"Yes," I said.

"Are you Tara Caimi?"

"Yes," I said again.

"*You're* Tara Caimi?" I stared at him in silence.

He introduced himself as the chaplain who also happened to be the father of a long-time friend and classmate of mine. After exchanging all the pleasantries I could muster, I wondered if he judged me for asking not to see him in the first place. I decided that he did, and rather than resume my fruitless effort to fall asleep, I was now forced to consider the concept of pride.

I had not wanted my name to appear in the newspaper, I admitted to myself, because I did not want the entire town to know how sick I was, or worse, to know *how* I was sick. I had no interest in receiving get-well balloons or flowers or, god forbid, visitors in my current state. I was melting from the inside out. It was hard enough to witness my own family witnessing that.

A philosophy professor in college once asked my class how each of us would prefer to die. I couldn't answer the question, but for some reason I later came up with my own variation of it. I chose, instead, to wonder about the most embarrassing way to die. Looking at my current situation, I felt certain that the melting method would rock the death charts to within the top twenty most humiliating approaches.

The chaplain could not have known about the plastic hat that rested upside-down in my personal hospital toilet or that underneath my not-so-fitted bed sheet lay an even less fitted plastic mat used under "normal" circumstances for the potty untrained or the otherwise continence challenged. Sure, it appeared I'd been sleeping in the middle of a weekday afternoon, but I was in a hospital. I had nothing to be ashamed of, I told myself. More importantly, I should not be called upon to make small talk while lying on my possible deathbed in a public hospital room. *How thoughtless and maybe even selfish of him to barge in like that when I specifically requested not to see him*, I fumed to the best of my weakened ability.

Prior to the chaplain experience, I believed I had lost all my pride, which, to my hospital-ridden self, seemed almost as useless as dignity. The chaplain experience changed that perspective. If it hadn't been for pride, I may have wanted to die from humiliation. As it was, my pride-inspired anger at the chaplain's imposition and subsequent judgment bolstered whatever strength I had left.

Had the chaplain really judged me? The answer didn't matter. Pride can certainly spark deception, self or otherwise directed, and it often rises from a deeply rooted basis of illusion, just like dignity. The difference is that pride, at least in my case, seemed to support the types of delusions that can serve to protect rather than tear down one's confidence. Not all my pride, I realized then, had gone down the toilet hat yet.

At night, the nurses took blood samples to monitor my condition. They came to my room every couple of hours, beginning at 11:00 p.m., each time extracting blood by poking into a new or a freshly healed hole with their needles, or taking my blood pressure, or checking my heart rate, or all of the above. At least my blood was flowing freely thanks to the IV, for which they also stabbed open a new puncture wound periodically.

Every morning, a doctor updated me on my condition. "You're ingesting the equivalent of this," he'd profess, drawing an imaginary line with his fingertip on an empty plastic soda bottle, "and you're eliminating twice that amount." There would be a pause.

I once described my pattern to the doctor, saying I felt strongest in the morning but progressively worse throughout the day. By evening, I retained the approximate strength of an overcooked spaghetti noodle. "I feel like my food is poisoning me," I once admitted, knowing it was outside the realm of possibility.

I was desperate and starving. I searched for food commercials on TV, salivating over images of Pizza Hut pizza and the double Whopper with cheese. When my doctor asked what I wanted to do when I got out of the hospital, I said, "I want to eat a bacon double cheeseburger."

"You don't eat bacon double cheeseburgers," he told me.

My mom started bringing me home-cooked meals. This covert activity contradicted the intake/outtake measuring approach, but I wasn't getting any better. The hospital food was barely identifiable, let alone edible. She could hardly watch my attempts to eat it.

Every few days I was allowed to walk down the hall for a shower. The nurses helped me wash so my IV didn't get wet. When I returned to the room, sometimes my dad would dry my hair like he did when I was a little girl. He'd set the dryer to low, slowly combing out the tangles until my chestnut-colored hair, which over the past few years had developed golden highlights, hung in loose waves around my face and over my shoulders. Devoid of sunlight for months, my skin had taken on a translucent quality, like skim milk, reminding me of the photograph I'd seen of myself as a baby, with the addition of a smattering of freckles across my cheeks and nose. My eyes, now ocean gray, rather than blue, once again resembled the porcelain doll eyes of the baby in that photograph.

The doctors ordered some upper GI tests and a CAT scan. As I sat in the wheelchair, awaiting my instructions, those ocean-gray eyes must have looked wide and terrified. The technician made small talk to ease my mind. She asked how old I was.

"Thirty," I told her, and her face went blank.

"I would have guessed eighteen," she said. Then she helped me out of the wheelchair to begin the procedures.

The stomach cramps hit me shortly after the CAT scan. I was still in my wheelchair, alone in the hallway and doubled over in pain, when my dad came in for one of his visits. I knew how it must have looked—his only daughter hunched in a wheelchair, dressed in only a hospital gown and attached to an IV, all skin and bones and hurt. I wished I could pretend it didn't hurt.

Dad wheeled me back to my room and by the time he left, the cramps had mercifully subsided. I watched *Animal Planet* on TV.

That night my mother stayed with me later than usual. One of the tests was intended to measure the length of time it took for substances to pass through my digestive tract, so food was off limits until the fluids I'd ingested that morning reached a certain point in my system. At 11:00 p.m., permission to eat had not yet been granted. I was weary from tests and feeble from lack of food, neither of which condition effectively suppressed the elimination problem. I maneuvered the IV stand into the bathroom to use the toilet hat facility. Moments later, I heard the nurse's voice.

"She's in the bathroom," my mother said, and I assumed the nurse would come back later.

Before I'd finished the thought, two quick knocks preceded the nurse's head poking from behind the now ajar bathroom door. "You can eat, you can eat!" She beamed at me. "What do you want for dinner?"

I looked up from my seated position. My mouth was no doubt open, but I found myself unable to speak.

"You just think about it, honey, and I'll come right back!"

I did appreciate the nurse's enthusiasm. I simply was unable to show it. To its credit, my ability to show appreciation had hung on a lot longer than my dignity had. I probably felt a tinge of guilt when I told the nurse, upon her return, that I wasn't hungry anymore and I just wanted to go to sleep. That's when I realized I wasn't angry or frustrated or even embarrassed by her breach of what I'd previously considered to be my privacy. *Where was my pride?* I wondered, sinking into bed amidst the familiar rustling of protective plastic under the sheets.

Around day seven, the doctors' faith in the stomach virus theory showed signs of wavering. An associate of my doctor came to my room to explain the next course of action. He was young—fresh out of med school, I presumed—and it looked to me like he struggled to maintain composure each time he uttered the word "diarrhea." To his misfortune, my case required liberal repetition of the word.

They were starting to eliminate possibilities, he told me, managing not to snicker. There was a very rare disease and almost no chance I had it, but they were going to rule out one potential cause at a time until the real culprit was revealed. They'd eliminate the least likely up front, then move on to those more probable. Again, he was sure I did not have this very rare disease, but procedure dictated they begin by testing for it.

A nurse handed me a two-inch stack of loose papers. "This is information on celiac disease," she said. "It's highly unlikely that this is what you have, but we'll be putting you on a special diet to be sure." I looked at the mountain of information on my lap, and for the first time,

I wanted to laugh. After everyone left the room, I picked up the first page. Celiac Disease; Gluten Intolerance; Gluten Sensitive Enteropathy; Malabsorption Syndrome; Nontropical Sprue...the list went on. I read three pages before agreeing conclusively with the doctor. I did not have that disease. People who had that disease could not eat anything. No pasta, no bread, no cake or cookies, no food with unknown origin, not to mention bacon double cheeseburgers. Those pages of information eradicated all food-related freedom. Not only did I love to eat, but also I was currently starving.

They put me on the diet, and my mom stopped bringing me buttered noodles in a thermos. Almost immediately, I showed signs of improvement. My doctor had been waiting for this glimmer of positive change, which afforded the window of opportunity he needed to carry out a plan. With measurable improvement, he'd release me from the hospital and arrange for a procedure to be performed by the gastroenterology specialist with whom he'd been in constant contact during my stay. As day eight showed more progress, my release was scheduled for day nine. The procedure turned out to be an endoscopy and a biopsy of my small intestine. It took place shortly after my release.

The results of the procedure would take a couple of weeks. I returned to work but not to any semblance of normalcy. My new diet consisted of bland meats, vegetables, fruits, potatoes, and rice. On this diet, my body inflated like the air mattress Nick and I had hooked up to our neighbor's battery-powered pump at the Wasatch State Park campgrounds two years prior. No amount of exercise curbed the supernatural growth spurt.

Two weeks after the procedure, I willed the phone on my desk to ring with the test results that would dictate my plans for the weekend. Before the stomach virus, I'd taken to tagging along with my parents and their friends on Friday nights to the local Italian restaurant. We'd drink Chianti and talk and laugh, and I'd devour mounds of angel hair pasta and eggplant Parmesan before retiring, satiated, home to bed.

After living away from my family for the past two years, these times together served as soul medicine. It was as much of an escape from the reality of my thirty-year-old life as it was an elixir—the strength of familial roots binding instinctively together to hold me up when I couldn't do it myself. Those Friday night dinners patched a hole in my heart. If only for a few brief hours each week, the pasta shared with family and friends filled me up.

That's why I stared at the telephone, willing it to ring on Friday afternoon at work. I needed those test results to tell me it was O.K. to eat pasta with my family. I needed to know I could fill myself up with it. When five o'clock came and the call with my test results did not, I decided to eat the pasta anyway.

It's possible I knew, on some subconscious level, that the evening at the Italian restaurant would be the last time I would ever order food without restriction in the company of family and friends. After a weekend of torturous purging, my confusion at the words, "You tested positive for celiac sprue," more likely resulted from the language used by the nurse on the telephone than the element of surprise at the reality of the situation—a reality that was no longer deniable.

I'd read the stack of papers the nurse had handed me in the hospital, along with other information I'd received after the endoscopy. I learned that celiac disease is an immune system disorder triggered by gluten, a protein in wheat, barley, and rye—grains used in everything from bread to pasta to cookies and cakes. When a person with celiac disease ingests gluten, her body attacks itself, destroying the parts of the intestine that absorb food and nutrients. The description I'd provided to my doctor in the hospital had been accurate, as impossible as it seemed. All this time, I'd been poisoning myself with the food I loved so much—the food I ate, not only for comfort but in order to stay alive. By trying to live just like everyone else, I had, in fact, been killing myself.

I have celiac disease, I repeated, pulling the notion back by a thread each time it drifted to the edge of acceptance. I wrapped it around my wrist like a childhood birthday balloon, determined not to let it get away. *This is my truth,* I thought. Unbeknownst to anyone, this truth had been with me forever.

33

NICK FOLLOWED THROUGH with plans to provide dog sled tours during the 2002 Winter Olympic Games. He called one evening to tell me he and the dog team were going to be featured on *The Today Show*. I relayed the pertinent portion of this news—that my puppies were going to be on TV—to my parents, Aunt Janet, and anyone else who might listen. When the episode aired, I barely recognized the team. My puppies were full-grown dogs and had replaced most of the original members. In standard fashion, Nick suffered no loss for words among the famed Katie Couric, Matt Lauer, and Al Roker—chatting with them in front of the television cameras as if they were old college buddies.

That spring, Nick returned to Pennsylvania to live with his father, bringing all the sled dogs and Little Cat with him. His father provided some land for a dog kennel, and I took the opportunity to reunite with my canine friends, traveling the twenty miles from my house to visit with Nick and the dogs as often as possible over the summer. The first time I entered the kennel, the puppies jumped on their hind legs and strained against their chains to reach me. I tried, with shamefully little success, to identify each one.

"They remember you," Nick said, though I scarcely believed him. "They wouldn't come out of their houses if they didn't."

"They're shy?" I asked scanning the kennel now populated primarily by this all blond litter. I saw signs of their mother in these adults and now recognized the button-like, teddy-bear eyes of another blond dog. Buster and Sandy had joined SnowDog Racing & Touring together the year after Nick and I arrived in Utah. Apparently, they'd taken more solace in each other's company than Nick and I had realized. Buster was the fastest dog in the kennel, Nick reminded me, which meant these puppies would be fast, too.

He would discover their true speed when he began his racing career in earnest the following winter. I said goodbye to my puppies a second time when they returned to Utah and to what I now accepted as their inevitable lives as working dogs. Nick and his team met with some success on the racing circuit that winter. Rather than celebrating, I looked forward to the following summer when I hoped to see them again, and I concentrated on healing my body, along with my heart, which had both been so sorely and recently damaged.

It would take many more years to complete the puzzle, putting into perspective the seemingly random pieces of my life that converged to form the path leading to my diagnosis in February 2002. I learned that celiac disease can be triggered by periods of illness or extreme stress and often goes undiagnosed because the symptoms match those of so many other conditions. If I hadn't struggled during those two years in Utah, my illness may have progressed undetected. Now I followed the prescription of a gluten-free diet, and the symptoms that had plagued me for thirty years subsided.

The next time I joined my family and their friends for dinner at the Italian restaurant, I ordered a salad rather than angel hair pasta, and my health fared much better through the weekend that followed.

A few months later, Grammie sat with me in the kitchen of my little yellow house, instructing as I mixed the gluten-free ingredients I'd purchased to mimic her renowned peanut butter Easter eggs.

"I'd like to give you all my recipes," she said as I stirred.

"You give too much away, Grammie."

"Oh, I'll never forget that story you wrote!" she laughed.

"The one where you sneak out at night in a trench coat and hat to secretly feed all the neighborhood dogs and hand money to strangers on street corners?"

"Your cousin's girlfriend laughed so hard, she cried."

"That's because it's not very far from the truth!"

"You wrote the whole story just sitting in the rocker one afternoon," she said. "I didn't know you could write like that."

"It's all I ever wanted to do," I said, hearing the words before I thought about what I was saying. I paused the mixer as the phrase echoed from the caverns of my mind. *It's all I ever wanted to do.*

The following Christmas, my mother and I altered the recipe for chicken divan to include a gluten-free version along with the regular meal. We organized a buffet-style layout, placing all gluten-free items in the breakfast nook to limit potential for cross-contamination of foods.

My new diet prohibited conventional participation in any situation involving people and food, and I learned to explain my condition with confidence. There was no alternative. There was no exception.

At that point I realized, since seventh grade cheerleading tryouts, I'd focused on finding ways to fit in. Through the years, I capitalized on my qualities that enhanced the potential for acceptance in peer groups, clubs, even careers, and I smothered those that did not. Rather than searching within for my path, I'd hitchhiked on those picked by others and accomplished with ease the appearance of personal choice. For the first time in my life, fitting in was no longer possible, which effectively shattered the pretense of trying. All this time, I'd maybe only been fooling myself.

When the Gardenias had called us their most "normal" friends, I'd felt something like a sense of accomplishment. It occurred to me now, the label wasn't bestowed as a compliment.

"Normal is bullshit," I said, feeling the words bubble up from an internal well and form in my mouth as I emptied them into the atmosphere.

I had a dream to follow. The next path I'd pursue would be my own. It would be all I ever wanted to do.

A Note on Celiac Disease

Twelve years after my diagnosis, I am still learning, and I know I will never stop. Celiac disease is an autoimmune disorder in which the small intestine is damaged when gluten is ingested, impairing the body's ability to digest food and absorb nutrients. Gluten is a protein found in grains including wheat, barley, and rye. These ingredients are hidden in more common foods than anyone who isn't forced to think about such things would imagine, such as soups and broth, seasonings, marinades, medications, and a host of processed food ingredients. Celiac disease can be triggered by stress, a viral infection, or any life-altering event[1]. Symptoms mirror those of many other illnesses and can include diarrhea, gas, bloating, lethargy, weakness, malnutrition, anemia, and hundreds more, many of which are caused by complications from the persistence of other symptoms. Though it is often misdiagnosed and even more often undiagnosed, celiac disease is not rare.

It is estimated that 1 in every 133 people in the United States has celiac disease[2]. An astounding 97% of those people remained undiagnosed as of 2006[3]. By 2014, the percentage of people with undiagnosed celiac disease had dropped to 83% [4].

Twelve years ago as I lay in the hospital bed, the doctor assured me celiac disease was rare. I've since learned that celiac disease is much more prevalent than was once thought; that the amount of gluten necessary to cause a negative reaction may vary per sensitivity level, current intestinal damage, and other individual factors; and that the disease is not always symptomatically perceptible.

Celiac disease is not rare. I will repeat this as many times as is necessary for the rest of my life. At the time I was diagnosed, it was not yet well accepted by the American medical profession. Finally, that is changing.

---

1   "What Is Celiac Disease?" *Celiac Disease Defined*. Celiac Support Association, n.d. Web. 13 Aug. 2014.

2   "Celiac Disease Facts & Figures." *NFCA Celiac Central*. National Foundation for Celiac Awareness, n.d. Web. 13 Aug. 2014.

3   p 3, Green H.R., Peter, M.D. and Jones, Rory. *Celiac Disease A Hidden Epidemic*. 1st ed., New York: HarperCollins, 2006.

4   "Celiac Disease Facts & Figures." *NFCA Celiac Central*. National Foundation for Celiac Awareness, n.d. Web. 13 Aug. 2014.

Resources

Mush: from sled dogs to celiac, the scenic detour of my life is intended to help raise awareness and to promote education and continued research of celiac disease. It is my hope that *Mush* also helps to promote the adoption of those Alaskan huskies out there in need of loving homes.

Resources I continue to rely on for current information on celiac disease include, but are not limited to, the following:

The Celiac Support Association at
www.csaceliacs.org/
Center for Celiac Research at
www.celiaccenter.org
The National Foundation for Celiac Awareness at
www.celiaccentral.org/
The University of Chicago Celiac Disease Center at
www.cureceliacdisease.org/

A compilation of local support groups listed by state across America can be found at www.celiac.com/articles/227/1/A-List-of-Local-Celiac-Disease-Support-GroupsChapters/Page1.html

I have found the following organizations and websites to be inspiring and helpful with regard to Alaskan husky rescue and resources:

Alaskan Husky Resources at
www.alaskan-husky-behavior.com/
The August Fund at
www.facebook.com/TheAugustFundforAlaskaRacingDogs

About the Author

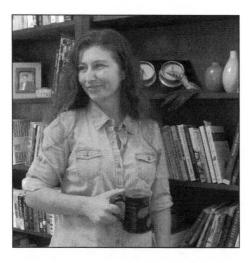

photo by Cristol Gregory

Tara Caimi is a freelance writer and editor living in State College, PA. Her work has been published in *The Writer's Chronicle*, *Oh Comely* magazine, *Fire & Knives* quarterly (sadly, out of print), the anthology *Whereabouts: Stepping out of Place*, and other journals and magazines. She is a member of the State College Celiac Support group, a sporadic volunteer at the no-kill animal shelter PAWS, and the adoptive mother of Kaela, a rescue husky mix. Visit her website at taracaimi.com.

Made in the USA
San Bernardino, CA
14 September 2016